LOW CHOLESTEROL DIET COOKBOOK FOR BEGINNERS 2024

Discover 101 Quick, Simple, and Healthy Recipes for Satisfying Meals to lower your cholesterol

+ 28-Day meal plan Bonus to get you started.

By: Verna R. Chapman

Copyright page

© 2024 Verna R. Chapman. All rights reserved. This book may not be reproduced, distributed, or transmitted in any form or by any means, including photocopying, recording, or other electronic or mechanical methods, without the publisher's prior written permission, with the exception of brief quotations included in critical reviews and specific other noncommercial uses allowed by copyright law.

Disclaimer

This book's content is meant to be used just for informative reasons; it is not meant to replace the counsel you receive from your doctor or other healthcare provider. Although the recipes and advice in this book are intended to promote a healthy lifestyle, each person's needs and circumstances are unique, so you should always speak with a healthcare provider before making any dietary or exercise changes. Any adverse effects or repercussions arising from using any recipes or suggestions in this book or from procedures followed after that are not the responsibility of the author or publisher. We have taken every precaution to guarantee that the content in this book is correct as of the publishing date. This book's author and publisher hereby explicitly disclaim any liability for negative consequences resulting from the use or use of its contents. Whenever you have concerns about your health or a medical condition, you should always seek the advice of your physician or another licensed healthcare professional. Pay attention to medical advice from professionals or put off getting it because of something you've read in this book.

HERE IS YOUR BONUS:

Here is a detailed 28-day meal plan to get you started with the LOW CHOLESTEROL DIET. All recipe processes for preparing the meals are discussed later in the guide.

Day 1

Breakfast: Low-Carb Blueberry Muffins

Lunch: Sheet-Pan Chicken Fajita Bowls

Dinner: Stuffed Zucchini Andalouse

Day 2

Breakfast: Date & Pine Nut Overnight Oatmeal

Lunch: Chicken Tagine

Dinner: Spicy Red Curry Beef & Rice

Day 3

Breakfast: Everything Bagel Avocado Toast

Lunch: Chipotle Chicken Quinoa Burrito Bowl

Dinner: Ground Beef & Potatoes Skillet

Day 4

Breakfast: Baked Banana-Nut Oatmeal Cups

Lunch: Slow-Cooker Chicken & White Bean Stew

Dinner: Cheesy Ground Beef & Cauliflower Casserole

Day 5

Breakfast: Smoked Salmon Breakfast Wraps

Lunch: Broccoli, Chicken Sausage & Orzo Skillet

Dinner: Italian-Style Beef & Pork Meatballs

Day 6

Breakfast: Cinnamon Streusel Rolls

Lunch: Lemon-Tahini Couscous with Chicken & Vegetables

Dinner: Slow-Cooker Balsamic Short Ribs

Day 7

Breakfast: Peanut Butter & Chia Berry Jam English Muffin

Lunch: Chicken Tinga Tostadas

Dinner: Beef Stir-Fry with Baby Bok Choy & Ginger

Day 8

Breakfast: Creamy Blueberry-Pecan Oatmeal

Lunch: One-Pot Spinach, Chicken Sausage & Feta Pasta

Dinner: Slow-Cooker Braised Beef with Carrots & Turnips

Day 9

Breakfast: Raspberry Yogurt Cereal Bowl

Lunch: Chicken & Vegetable Penne with Parsley-Walnut Pesto

Dinner: Rosemary & Garlic-Basted Sirloin Steak

Day 10

Breakfast: Rhubarb Oat Muffins

Lunch: Slow-Cooker Chicken & Chickpea Soup

Dinner: Skillet Steak with Mushroom Sauce

Day 11

Breakfast: Apple Cinnamon Chia Pudding

Lunch: Ancho Chicken Breast with Black Beans, Bell Peppers & Scallions

Dinner: Slow-Cooked Beef with Carrots & Cabbage

Day 12

Breakfast: Almond-Matcha Green Smoothie Bowl

Lunch: Slow-Cooker Chicken & Orzo with Tomatoes & Olives

Dinner: Beef & Bean Sloppy Joes

Day 13

Breakfast: Peanut Butter Protein Overnight Oats

Lunch: Chicken & Cucumber Lettuce Wraps with Peanut Sauce

Dinner: Slow-Cooker Beef Stroganoff

Day 14

Breakfast: Low-Carb Blueberry Muffins

Lunch: Slow-Cooker Chicken with Rosemary & Mushrooms over Linguine

Dinner: Scallion-Ginger Beef & Broccoli

Day 15

Breakfast: Date & Pine Nut Overnight Oatmeal

Lunch: Chicken & Sun-Dried Tomato Orzo

Dinner: Tater Tot Casserole with Beef, Corn & Zucchini

Day 16

Breakfast: Everything Bagel Avocado Toast

Lunch: Stuffed Zucchini Andalouse

Dinner: One-Pot Garlicky Shrimp & Spinach

Day 17

Breakfast: Baked Banana-Nut Oatmeal Cups

Lunch: Walnut-Rosemary Crusted Salmon

Dinner: Slow-Cooker Braised Beef with Carrots & Turnips

Day 18

Breakfast: Smoked Salmon Breakfast Wraps

Lunch: Seasoned Cod

Dinner: Slow-Cooker Chicken & Chickpea Soup

Day 19

Breakfast: Cinnamon Streusel Rolls

Lunch: Salmon with Lemon-Herb Orzo & Broccoli

Dinner: Beef Stir-Fry with Baby Bok Choy & Ginger

Day 20

Breakfast: Peanut Butter & Chia Berry Jam English Muffin

Lunch: Italian Mussels & Pasta

Dinner: Cheesy Ground Beef & Cauliflower Casserole

Day 21

Breakfast: Creamy Blueberry-Pecan Oatmeal

Lunch: Sheet-Pan Chili-Lime Salmon with Potatoes & Peppers

Dinner: Italian-Style Beef & Pork Meatballs

Day 22

Breakfast: Raspberry Yogurt Cereal Bowl

Lunch: Spicy Jerk Shrimp

Dinner: Slow-Cooker Balsamic Short Ribs

Day 23

Breakfast: Rhubarb Oat Muffins

Lunch: Provençal Baked Fish with Roasted Potatoes & Mushrooms

Dinner: Ground Beef & Potatoes Skillet

Day 24

Breakfast: Apple Cinnamon Chia Pudding

Lunch: Skillet Gnocchi with Shrimp & Asparagus

Dinner: Chicken & Vegetable Penne with Parsley-Walnut Pesto

Day 25

Breakfast: Almond-Matcha Green Smoothie Bowl

Lunch: Herby Fish with Wilted Greens & Mushrooms

Dinner: Slow-Cooker Chicken with Rosemary & Mushrooms over Linguine

Day 26

Breakfast: Peanut Butter Protein Overnight Oats

Lunch: Oven-Fried Fish & Chips

Dinner: Beef & Bean Sloppy Joes

Day 27

Breakfast: Low-Carb Blueberry Muffins

Lunch: Shrimp-Stuffed Pasta Shells

Dinner: Slow-Cooked Beef with Carrots & Cabbage

Day 28

Breakfast: Date & Pine Nut Overnight Oatmeal

Lunch: Peppery Barbecue-Glazed Shrimp with Vegetables & Orzo

Dinner: Slow-Cooker Beef Stroganoff

ABOUT THE AUTHOR

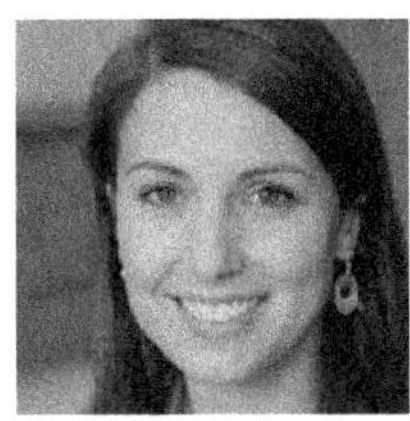 **Chef Verna R. Chapman** enthusiastically supports a healthy diet and way of life. She has devoted her career to turning classic recipes into heart-friendly treats, as she strongly believes in preparing nourishing meals that unite people. Growing up in a household where cooking was valued as an art and a way of life, Verna fell in love at an early age with preparing meals that unite people. Her culinary adventures have brought her from amateur kitchens to commercial kitchens, where she has refined her culinary techniques and expanded her understanding of food and nutrition. This is based on Verna's perception of healthy eating, which resulted from personal experience and the need to improve her life.

For several years, she tried various ingredients and cooking techniques that created tasty meals that benefited her health. This strategy makes her an authority in the culinary world, especially for those who wish to adopt a healthy diet. Apart from being a professional chef, Verna is also a happy wife. She likes involving her family in a healthy lifestyle, believing that delicious food is the key to a happy life. Her husband is usually with her in the kitchen, and they try out new recipes to prepare food for their family.

In her books and recipes she is developing, Verna encourages others to lead a healthy life. Thus, the title "LOW CHOLESTEROL DIET COOKBOOK FOR BEGINNERS 2024" carries out her mission of specializing in making healthy meals for the heart willingly obtained by anyone. Whether you have been cooking for years or have just begun this journey, with the help of Verna's recipes, you can create tasty and healthy dishes that will allow you to improve your health and enjoy every bite. Verna R. Chapman would like to take your hand and lead you to improved health while enjoying every bite. With her help, you can prepare delicious food at home that nourishes your heart and soul.

Table of contents

Introduction

Welcome to the "LOW CHOLESTEROL DIET COOKBOOK FOR BEGINNERS 2024" Few things are more critical in the quest for a healthier living than our decisions regarding our diet. This book is meant to guide your journey toward improved heart health; it includes delicious and nutritious recipes that are simple to follow. Finding the time to cook healthy meals might be challenging in today's fast-paced world. Preparing gratifying meals that lower cholesterol levels and nourish the body with the correct advice is feasibly the proper advice. This book is designed to suit the needs of all cooks, from beginners to seasoned pros searching for new ideas. These pages contain a variety of recipes that are meant to be easy to prepare and quick to make so you can quickly create delicious dinners. Every recipe, from filling dinners designed to robust brunches, is created with your heart health in mind.

These recipes help you navigate a healthy lifestyle using nutrient-rich products and mindful cooking methods. They also taste fantastic lifestyle. However, this book is more than just a compilation of recipes; it's a manual for comprehending the function of cholesterol in our bodies and how food choices can enhance heart health. You'll discover how to make wise dietary choices by reading insightful articles and using helpful advice, eventually enabling you to lead a longer, healthier life. "LOW CHOLESTEROL DIET COOKBOOK FOR BEGINNERS 2024" is therefore here to accompany you every step of the way, whether your goals are to lower cholesterol, improve heart health, or simply enjoy delectable meals that nourish the body and spirit.

Here is to adopting a better lifestyle!

How to Use This Book

This book aims to assist you in transitioning to a heart-healthy diet plan and offers delicious recipes for maintaining low cholesterol. Here's how to make the most of it:

1. **Start with the Basics:** Firstly, familiarize yourself with the essential sections of the site to gain a comprehensive understanding of the benefits of a low-cholesterol diet for your body. The following foundation will help you make the right choices as you progress along this path.
2. **Follow the 28-Day Meal Plan:** The book offers a 28-day meal plan as a starting point. It is a practical method for introducing healthy recipes to your everyday diet pattern. The meal plan includes all of the day's meals, ensuring a balanced diet.
3. **Check out the recipes**: The different types of meals distinguish each chapter, and each chapter contains the following information:
- *Chapter 3: Breakfast:* Kickstart your morning meal with some heart-friendly

recipes that you can try at home, including low-carb blueberry muffins, date and pine nuts overnight oatmeal, and avocado toast.

- *Chapter 4: Poultry:* These are some mouth-watering dishes that you can prepare using poultry products, such as sheet-pan chicken fajita bowls, chicken tagine, slow-cooker chicken, and white bean stew.
- *Chapter 5: Meat* For those who prefer large meat dishes, there are options such as stuffed zucchini and potatoes, spicy red curry beef and rice, and ground beef and potato skillet.
- *Chapter 6: Seafood:* Savor seafood recipes like Lemon-Tahini Couscous with Chicken and Vegetables, Italian Mussels and Pasta, and Scallion-Ginger Beef and Broccoli.
- *Chapter 7: Vegetarian:* Some options can be the Baked Banana-Nut Oatmeal Cups, Smoked Salmon Breakfast Wraps, Creamy Blueberry-Pecan Oatmeal, and more.
- *Chapter 8: Desserts*: Cravings for sweets can be satisfied via skinny desserts such as Rhubarb Oat Muffins, Cinnamon Streusel Rolls, and Peanut Butter Protein Overnight Oats.
- *Chapter 9: Smoothies:* Quench your thirst with wholesome smoothies, such as the almond-matcha green smoothie bowl and the peanut butter protein overnight oats, among others, which you will find in many chapters of the book.
- *Chapter 10 snacks and side*: Snacks and side dishes include recipes like the Apple Cinnamon Chia Pudding, Homemade

Pizza Sauce, and the Almond-Matcha Green Smoothie Bowl.

4. **Use the Tips and Tricks:** Here are important tips and suggestions about what, how, and when to prepare, what to replace an ingredient with, and how to cook healthier. We aim to enhance your cooking experience and maximize its potential.

5. **Track Your Progress:** We recommend paying close attention to the fluctuations in cholesterol levels and overall health, in addition to the diet. To properly monitor your progress and make necessary changes, we advise you to maintain a food diary.

6. **Learn the essentials:** The following sections comprise the completed book:

- *Understanding Cholesterol and Heart Health:* Here you will find out what beneficial cholesterol is and what harmful cholesterol is, what disorders high cholesterol levels entail, and what is advantageous about a low cholesterol diet.
- *Managing Cholesterol Levels:* Learn about the changes you need to make in your routines, diet, and regular health check-ups that are essential when you have high cholesterol.
- *Foods to Eat and Foods to Avoid:* Consult and obtain a list of foods that fit into a low-cholesterol diet, as well as those that should be avoided.
- *Understanding Cholesterol Metrics:* Gain a thorough understanding of how cholesterol information affects your health.

Understanding Cholesterol and Heart Health

Cholesterol, a waxy compound in the blood, is vital for cell growth, hormone production, and digestion. However, high cholesterol levels can have major health consequences, particularly for your cardiovascular system. Understanding how cholesterol impacts your health is the first step toward adopting healthier food decisions.

Good vs. Bad Cholesterol

Lipoproteins carry cholesterol throughout the bloodstream. There are two sorts that you should be aware of:

- *Lower-Density Lipoprotein (LDL)*: High levels of LDL, sometimes known as "bad" cholesterol, can cause the formation of fatty deposits in your arteries, raising your risk of heart disease and stroke.
- *High-Density Lipoproteins (HDL),* sometimes known as "good" cholesterol, transport cholesterol from your arteries to the liver, where it is processed and eliminated from the body.

Health Risks Associated with High Cholesterol

- *Atherosclerosis:* When cholesterol and other compounds accumulate in the artery walls, plaques form, causing the arteries to narrow and stiffen, reducing blood flow.
- *Coronary Artery Disease (CAD):* Plaques can restrict blood flow to the heart muscle, causing chest pain and heart attacks if they rupture and form a clot.
- *Stroke:* Reduced or obstructed blood supply to the brain caused by narrowed or clogged arteries can lead to a stroke.
- *Peripheral Artery Disease (PAD):* Plaques in the arteries of the limbs, particularly the legs, can cause pain, movement problems, and an increased risk of infection.
- *High Blood Pressure:* High cholesterol causes narrower arteries, which forces the heart to work harder to pump blood through them, resulting in high blood pressure.
- *Metabolic Syndrome:* A combination of high cholesterol, high blood pressure, high blood sugar, and extra abdominal fat raises the risk of heart disease, stroke, and diabetes.

Benefits of a Low Cholesterol Diet

A low-cholesterol diet has various health benefits:

- Lowering LDL levels reduces the risk of heart attacks and strokes and improves overall heart health.

- A diet high in heart-healthy foods helps enhance blood pressure and circulation.
- Promotes weight management: Many low-cholesterol foods are low in calories and high in nutrients, which helps with weight control.

Managing Cholesterol Levels

Make lifestyle adjustments to regulate cholesterol levels and lower the risk of linked health problems. Here are some of the ways to reduce cholesterol levels:

- *Healthy Diet:* Eat meals low in saturated and trans fats. Include more fruits, vegetables, whole grains, lean proteins, and healthy fats such as nuts and olive oil.
- *Regular exercise* raises HDL cholesterol while lowering LDL cholesterol and triglycerides.
- *Maintain a Healthy Weight:* Being overweight or obese might increase LDL cholesterol while decreasing HDL cholesterol.
- *Limit Alcohol Consumption:* Drinking too much alcohol can raise triglycerides and increase the risk of heart disease.
- *Medication:* In some circumstances, lifestyle changes alone are insufficient, and medicines may be needed to assist in managing cholesterol levels.

Monitoring and Regular Checkups

Regular cholesterol screenings and health checkups are required for early detection and treatment of high cholesterol. Understanding your cholesterol levels and working with your doctor to keep them healthy can significantly lower your risk of heart disease and improve your general health.

Adopting a heart-healthy lifestyle and making smart dietary choices can help you manage your cholesterol and safeguard your cardiovascular health.

Understanding Cholesterol Metrics

To manage cholesterol effectively, it's important to understand your cholesterol metrics:

Total Cholesterol: The overall amount of cholesterol in your blood.

Desirable: Less than 200 mg/dL

Borderline high: 200-239 mg/dL

High: 240 mg/dL and above

LDL Cholesterol:

Optimal: Less than 100 mg/dL

Near optimal/above optimal: 100-129 mg/dL

Borderline high: 130-159 mg/dL

High: 160-189 mg/dL

Very high: 190 mg/dL and above

HDL Cholesterol:

Low (and risky): Less than 40 mg/dL for men, less than 50 mg/dL for women

High (and protective): 60 mg/dL and above

Triglycerides: Another type of fat in the blood.

Normal: Less than 150 mg/dL

Borderline high: 150-199 mg/dL

High: 200-499 mg/dL

Very high: 500 mg/dL and above

Foods to Eat and Foods to Avoid

Foods to Eat:

- Fruits and vegetables
- Whole grains
- Lean proteins (poultry, fish, legumes)
- Nuts and seeds
- Healthy fats (olive oil, avocado)

Foods to Avoid:

- Saturated fats (butter; fatty portions of meat)
- Trans fats (margarine and fried meals)
- Processed meats (sausage and bacon)
- High-cholesterol foods (organ meats and full-fat dairy)

Shopping List

Here is a shopping list to help you get started with the 28 meals:

Fruits and Vegetables

- Blueberries (fresh or frozen)
- Dates
- Pine nuts
- Avocados
- Bananas
- Apples
- Raspberries
- Rhubarb
- Zucchini
- Broccoli
- Baby Bok Choy
- Spinach
- Carrots
- Turnips
- Peppers (red, green, yellow)
- Onions (yellow, red)
- Garlic
- Fresh parsley
- Fresh basil
- Fresh cilantro
- Lemon
- Lime
- Mushrooms (cremini, shiitake)
- Kale
- Tomatoes (plum, cherry, fire-roasted canned)
- Artichoke hearts (frozen or canned)
- Cucumbers (English, regular)
- Scallions
- Baby spinach

- Snow peas or snap peas

- Fresh dill

- Radishes

- Fresh ginger

Proteins

- Chicken breasts

- Chicken thighs (bone-in, skinless)

- Chicken tenders

- Chicken sausage

- Ground chicken breast

- Ground beef (90% lean)

- Ground pork

- Beef tenderloin

- Beef short ribs

- Sirloin steak

- Beef stew meat

- Pork loin

- Salmon (smoked, fresh)

- Cod

- Shrimp

- Mussels

- Eggs

- Greek yogurt (nonfat plain)

- Cheddar cheese (extra-sharp)

- Feta cheese (reduced-fat)

- Parmesan cheese (grated)

- Romano cheese (finely shredded)

- Ricotta cheese

- Cream cheese (light)

- Cottage cheese

- Light sour cream

Grains and Legumes

- Old-fashioned rolled oats

- Steel-cut oats

- Whole-wheat bread

- Whole-wheat English muffins

- Whole-wheat flour

- Whole-wheat pasta (penne, rotini, linguine)

- Whole-wheat orzo

- Brown rice

- Quinoa

- Couscous (whole-wheat pearl)

- Panko breadcrumbs (preferably whole-wheat)

- Cannellini beans (dried)

- Black beans (canned, low-sodium)

- Garbanzo beans (canned)

- Pinto beans (canned)
- Refried beans (low-sodium)
- Lentils (brown)
- Chickpeas (dried, canned)
- Mini shredded-wheat cereal
- Farro
- Gnocchi

Pantry Staples

- Almond flour
- Coconut flour
- Baking powder
- Baking soda
- Light brown sugar
- Avocado oil
- Olive oil (extra-virgin)
- Coconut oil
- Chia seeds
- Peanut butter (natural, powdered)
- Pure maple syrup
- Tomato paste
- Canned tomatoes (no-salt-added diced, fire-roasted diced)
- Tomato sauce (no-salt-added)
- Coconut milk (light)
- Chicken broth (low-sodium)
- Vegetable broth (low-sodium)
- Fish sauce
- Soy sauce (low-sodium)
- Worcestershire sauce
- Balsamic vinegar
- Red wine vinegar
- Apple cider vinegar
- White vinegar
- Honey
- Mustard (Dijon, yellow)
- Nutritional yeast
- Vanilla extract
- Pure pumpkin puree
- Baking cocoa (unsweetened)
- Gelatin (unflavored)
- Sea salt
- Kosher salt
- Ground black pepper
- Cayenne pepper
- Crushed red pepper
- Ground cumin

- Ground cinnamon
- Ground turmeric
- Ground paprika
- Ground ginger
- Ground coriander
- Ground cardamom
- Ground cloves
- Ground nutmeg
- Smoked paprika
- Chili powder
- Italian seasoning
- Herbes de Provence
- Dried basil
- Dried thyme
- Dried oregano
- Bay leaves
- Canned chipotle peppers in adobo sauce

Dairy and Alternatives

- Skim milk
- Low-fat milk
- Unsweetened almond milk
- Soy milk (or other plant-based milk)
- Low-fat yogurt
- Reduced-fat cheese
- Light cream cheese spread
- Light sour cream

Other

- Pine nuts
- Walnuts
- Almonds (sliced, chopped, toasted)
- Pecans (chopped, toasted)
- Pumpkin seeds
- Sunflower seeds
- Poppy seeds
- Flaxseeds
- Sesame seeds
- Dark chocolate chips
- Mini chocolate chips
- Dried cranberries
- Raisins
- Medjool dates
- Dried apricots
- Sun-dried tomatoes (not oil-packed)
- Black olives (pitted, quartered)
- Green olives (pitted, quartered)
- Kalamata olives (pitted, chopped)

Additional Items for Specific Recipes

- Puff pastry sheets (frozen)

- Whole-wheat tortillas

- Tortilla chips

- English muffins

- Muffin liners

BREAKFAST

Low-Carb Blueberry Muffins

Prep Time: 15 mins **Additional Time:** 45 mins **Total Time:** 1 hr.

Servings: 12   **Yield:** 12 muffins

Ingredients

1 ¾ cups almond flour

¼ cup coconut flour

1 tablespoon baking powder

¼ teaspoon baking soda

¼ teaspoon salt

1 cup blueberries

3 large eggs

½ cup reduced-fat milk

⅓ cup plus 2 tablespoons light brown sugar

¼ cup avocado oil

1 ½ teaspoons vanilla extract

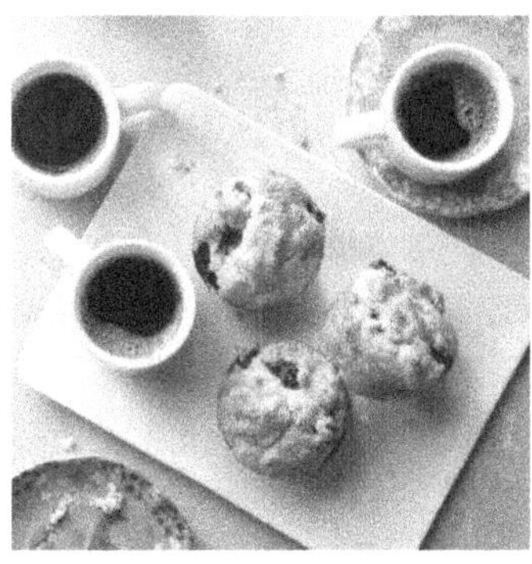

Directions

Preheat oven to 350 degrees Fahrenheit. Coat a muffin tin liberally with cooking spray.

Combine almond flour, coconut flour, baking powder, baking soda, and salt in a large bowl.

Add the blueberries and stir to coat. In a medium bowl, whisk together the eggs, milk, brown sugar, oil, and vanilla. Add to the dry ingredients and mix to blend. Divide the batter evenly among the muffin cups (about 1/4 cup per cup).

Bake muffins until gently browned and a toothpick inserted in the center comes out clean, about 20-25 minutes. Allow to cool in the pan on a wire rack for 20 minutes. Run a knife around the edges, then remove from the tin to cool fully.

Nutrition Facts (per serving)

204	15g	15g	6g
Calories	Fat	Carbs	Protein

Date & Pine Nut Overnight Oatmeal

Prep Time: 10 mins   **Additional Time:** 7 hrs. 50 mins   **Total Time:** 8 hrs.

Servings: 1   **Yield:** 1 cup

Ingredients

- ½ cup old-fashioned rolled oats
- ½ cup water
- Pinch of salt
- 2 tablespoons chopped dates
- 1 tablespoon toasted pine nuts
- 1 teaspoon honey
- ¼ teaspoon ground cinnamon

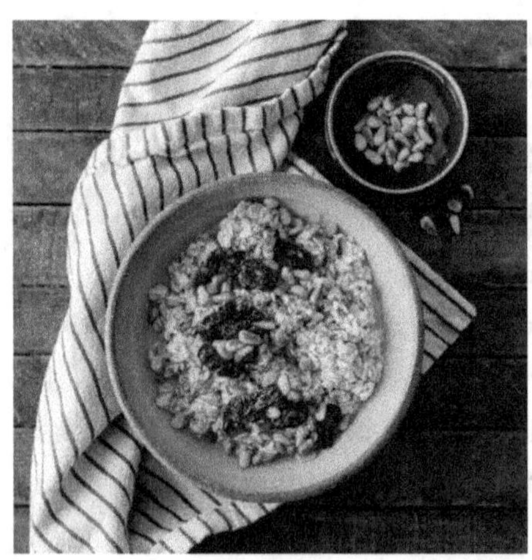

Directions

Mix oats, water, and salt in a bowl or container. Stir well. Cover and refrigerate overnight.

You can either boil the oats or consume them cold. Garnish with dates, pine nuts, honey, and cinnamon.

Tips:

For those with celiac disease or gluten sensitivity, use "gluten-free" oats to avoid cross-contamination with wheat and barley.

To make ahead: When preparing oatmeal the night before, measure, toast, and cut topping ingredients.

Nutrition Facts (per serving)

282	Calories
9g	Fat
48g	Carbs
7g	Protein

Everything Bagel Avocado Toast

Prep Time: 5 mins

Total Time: 5 mins

Servings: 1

Yield: 1 toast

Ingredients

¼ medium avocado, mashed

1 slice whole-grain bread, toasted

2 teaspoons of everything bagel seasoning

Pinch of flaky sea salt (such as Maldon)

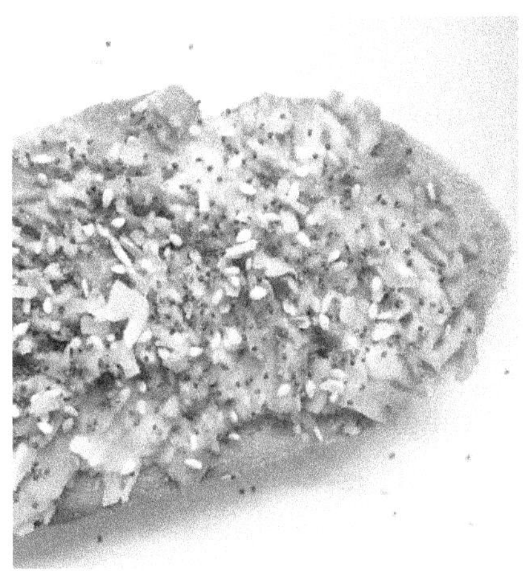

Directions

Spread avocado onto bread. Sprinkle with spice and salt.

Nutrition Facts (per serving)

172	Calories
10g	Fat
18g	Carbs
5g	Protein

Baked Banana-Nut Oatmeal Cups

Prep Time: 15 mins

Additional Time: 35 mins

Total Time: 50 mins   **Servings:** 12   **Yield:** 12 muffins

Here's How I Made This Recipe to Be Healthy and Diabetes-Friendly:

High levels of added sugar can negatively affect blood sugar. I reduced brown sugar to ⅓ cup and sweetened oatmeal cups with bananas, cinnamon, and vanilla flavors. Traditional muffin recipes generally contain double the amount of sugar, making them more of a treat than a nutritious breakfast or snack.

Rolled oats include soluble fiber, which helps regulate blood sugar levels and increase fullness. Each muffin contains 1/4 cup of rolled oats, resulting in 3 grams of fiber per serving.

The muffin tin serves as both a cooking vessel and a convenient storage container for individual oatmeal cups. This relieves the burden of measuring, making snacking or breakfast easier, and helps you avoid overeating or undereating.

Ingredients

3 cups rolled oats (see Tip)

1 ½ cups low-fat milk

2 ripe bananas, mashed (about 3/4 cup)

⅓ cup packed brown sugar

2 large eggs, lightly beaten

1 teaspoon baking powder

1 teaspoon ground cinnamon

1 teaspoon vanilla extract

½ teaspoon salt

½ cup toasted chopped pecans

Directions

Preheat the oven to 375°F. Coat the muffin tray with cooking spray.

Combine oats, milk, bananas, brown sugar, eggs, baking powder, cinnamon, vanilla, and salt in a large basin. Fold in pecans.

Divide the mixture between the muffin cups (approximately 1/3 cup each).

Bake for approximately 25 minutes, or until a toothpick inserted into the center comes clean.

Allow 10 minutes to cool in the pan before transferring to a wire rack. Serve warm or at room temperature.

Tip

People with celiac disease or gluten sensitivity should use "gluten-free" oats, as they are frequently cross-contaminated with wheat and barley.

Nutrition Facts (per serving)

176	Calories
6g	Fat
26g	Carbs
5g	Protein

Smoked Salmon Breakfast Wraps

Prep Time: 20 mins   **Total Time:** 20 mins

Servings: 4   **Yield:** 4 servings

Ingredients

⅓ cup light cream cheese spread

1 tablespoon snipped fresh chives

1 teaspoon finely shredded lemon peel

1 tablespoon lemon juice

4 6 to 7-inch whole wheat flour tortillas

3 ounces thinly sliced, smoked salmon (lox-style), cut into strips

1 small zucchini, trimmed

4 Lemon wedge

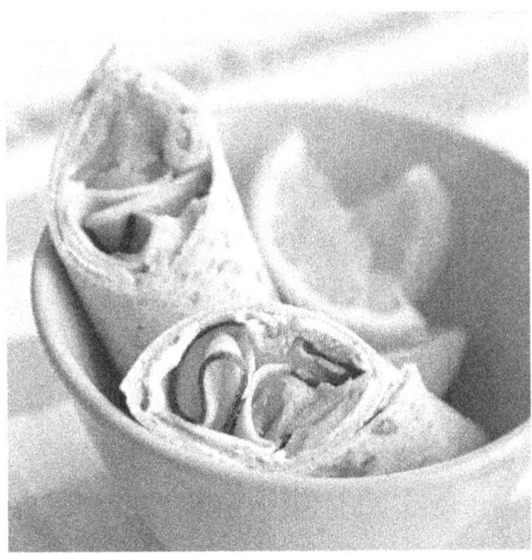

Directions

In a small bowl, mix cream cheese, chives, lemon peel, and lemon juice until smooth.

Spread equally over tortillas, leaving a half-inch border around the borders.

Arrange salmon on the bottom half of each tortilla. To create zucchini ribbons, draw a sharp vegetable peeler lengthwise down the zucchini and cut very thin slices.

Place the zucchini ribbons on top of the fish.

Roll tortillas from the bottom up. Cut in half. If preferred, serve with lemon wedges.

Nutrition Facts (per serving)

124	Calories
6g	Fat
14g	Carbs
12g	Protein

Cinnamon Streusel Rolls

Prep Time: 45 mins   **Additional Time:** 2 hrs.   **Total Time:** 2 hrs. 45 mins

Servings: 15   **Yield:** 15 rolls

Ingredients

1 cup fat-free milk plus 2 to 3 teaspoons, divided

2 teaspoons packed brown sugar (see Tip)

¼ cup tub-style 60-70% vegetable oil spread, divided

1 teaspoon salt

¼ cup warm water (110 to 115 degrees F)

1 package active dry yeast

¼ cup refrigerated or frozen egg product, thawed, or 1 egg, lightly beaten

4-4 1/2 cups all-purpose flour (see Tip)

½ cup rolled oats, toasted (see Tip)

2 teaspoons ground cinnamon

¼ cup chopped pecans, toasted (see Tip)

⅓ cup light sour cream

¼ cup powdered sugar

¼ teaspoon vanilla extract

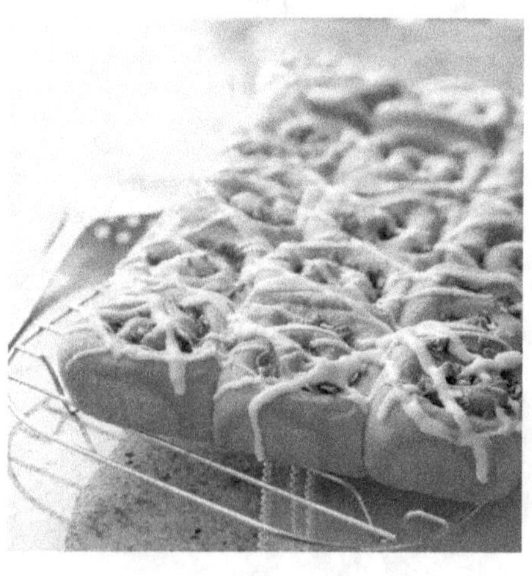

Directions

Put 1 cup of milk, 2 tablespoons of vegetable oil spread, brown sugar, and salt in a small pot. Warm up until hot (110 to 115 degrees F). Put away.

Put the yeast and warm water in a big bowl. Ten minutes should pass. The egg and milk mixture should be added to the yeast mixture.

Mix the flour substitute (if you're using it; see Tip) with as much of the extra all-purpose flour as you can with a wooden spoon.

Move the dough to an area that has been lightly floured. Use the rest of the flour to knead the dough until it is slightly soft, smooth, and stretchy (3 to 5 minutes).

Make a ball out of the dough. If you want to grease the surface, put the food in a bowl and turn it once to cover it. It will double in size in about an hour if you cover it and leave it somewhere warm.

Press the dough down. Spread out on a surface that has been lightly floured. Set it aside for 10 minutes with the lid on.

In the meantime, butter a 13x9-inch baking pan and set it away. Mix the oats and cinnamon together in a medium bowl.

Use your fingers to spread the last two tablespoons of vegetable oil out. In a medium bowl, mix the oats and cinnamon together.

The dough should be rolled out into a 15x8-inch square. Leave a 1-inch gap on one of the long sides and sprinkle with the nut mixture. Start with the filling on the long side and roll up into a spiral.

 Close the seam by pinching the dough together. Then, cut it into 15 uniform pieces. Put the pieces in the baking pan with the cut sides facing up. Let it rise in a warm place for about 30 minutes, or until it's almost doubled in size.

Warm the oven up to 375 degrees F. After 25 to 30 minutes, the bread should be golden. For 5 minutes, let it cool in the pan on a wire rack.

To make a drizzle, mix together sour cream, powdered sugar, vanilla, and 2 to 3 teaspoons of milk.

Take the rolls out of the pan. Add frosting on top. Warm up and serve.

Tips

You can use Sweet Low Brown or Sugar Twin Granulated Brown instead of sugar if you need to. To use the amount that is equal to two teaspoons of brown sugar, follow the directions on the package. Nutrition facts for one serving of the replacement are the same as those below, but it has 189 calories, 31 grams of carbs, and 198 mg of sodium.

For every 2 cups of all-purpose flour, you can use whole-wheat flour, white whole-wheat flour, whole-wheat pastry flour, or whole-grain oat flour instead. Different types of flour have different amounts of calories, carbs, fiber, and protein per serving. Whole-wheat flour has 189 calories, 32 grams of carbs, 3 grams of fiber, and 6 grams of protein. White whole-wheat flour has 188 calories, 198 milligrams of sodium, 32 grams of carbs, and 6 grams of protein. White whole-wheat pastry flour has 194 calories, 198 milligrams of sodium, 32 grams of carbs, and 3 grams of fiber. Whole-grain oat flour has 200 calories, 6 grams of fat, 198 milligrams of sodium, 31 grams of carbs, and 6 grams of protein.

Place the oats in a large pan. Cook them over medium-low heat, stirring them often, for 4 to 5 minutes, or until they are lightly toasted. Put nuts in a small baking pan lined with parchment paper to toast them. Let it bake at 350°F for 5 to 10 minutes, or until it turns brown. Once or twice, shake the pan.

Nutrition Facts (per serving)

194	Calories
5g	Fat
33g	Carbs
5g	Protein

Peanut Butter & Chia Berry Jam English Muffin

Cook Time: 10 mins   **Total Time:** 10 mins

Servings: 1   **Yield:** 1 serving

Ingredients

½ cup unsweetened mixed frozen berries

2 teaspoons chia seeds

2 teaspoons natural peanut butter

1 whole-wheat English muffin, toasted

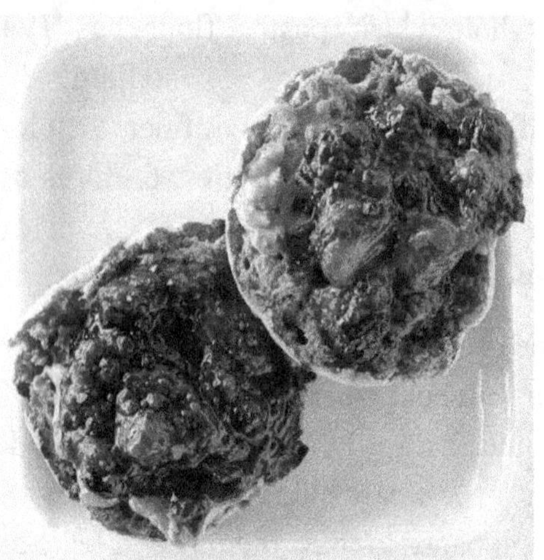

Directions

Use a medium-sized bowl that can go in the microwave and heat the berries for 30 seconds. Then toss them around and microwave for another 30 seconds.

Add the chia seeds and mix them in.

Toast an English muffin and put peanut butter on it. Add the berry-chia mix on top.

Nutrition Facts (per serving)

262	Calories
9g	Fat
41g	Carbs
10g	Protein

Creamy Blueberry-Pecan Oatmeal

Cook Time: 10 mins   **Total Time:** 10 mins

Servings: 1   **Yield:** 1 serving

Ingredients

1 cup water

Pinch of salt

½ cup old-fashioned rolled oats

½ cup blueberries, fresh or frozen, thawed

2 tablespoons nonfat plain Greek yogurt

1 tablespoon toasted chopped pecans

2 teaspoons pure maple syrup

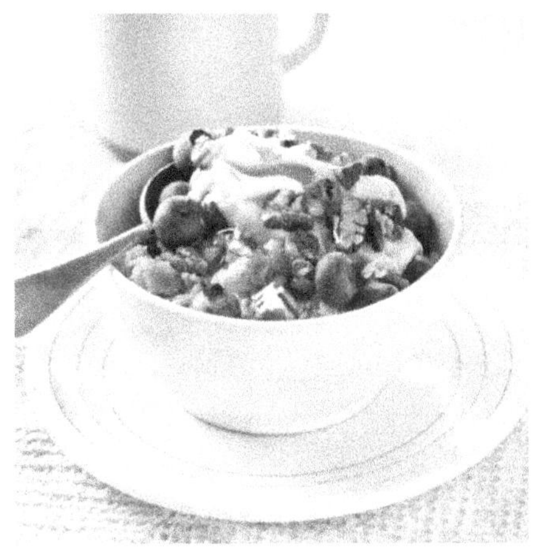

Directions

In a small pot, bring water and salt to a boil.

Add the oats and stir them in. Then lower the heat to medium and let it boil, stirring every so often, for about 5 minutes, or until the liquid is gone.

Take it off the heat, cover it, and let it sit for two to three minutes. Blueberries, yogurt, nuts, and syrup should be put on top.

Tips

Overnight oatmeal variation: In a jar or bowl, combine 1/2 cup old-fashioned rolled oats, 1/2 cup water, and a teaspoon of salt. Cover and store in the refrigerator overnight. Add toppings in the morning. Eat cold or heat up. Makes about one cup.

Steel-cut oats recipe variation: Bring 1 cup water and a pinch of salt to a boil in a small saucepan. Add 1/3 cup steel-cut oats, reduce heat to a low simmer, cover, and cook for 15 to 20 minutes, stirring regularly, until most of the liquid is absorbed. Remove from heat and allow stand for 2 to 3 minutes, covered. Add the desired toppings. Makes about one cup.

People suffering from celiac disease or gluten sensitivity should buy oats labeled "gluten-free," as oats are frequently cross-contaminated with wheat and barley

	291	Calories
	8g	Fat

Nutrition Facts (per serving)

49g	Carbs
9g	Protein

Raspberry Yogurt Cereal Bowl

Prep Time: 5 mins   **Total Time:** 5 mins

Servings: 1   **Yield:** 1 serving

Ingredients

1 cup nonfat plain yogurt

½ cup mini shredded-wheat cereal

¼ cup fresh raspberries

2 teaspoons mini chocolate chips

1 teaspoon pumpkin seeds

¼ teaspoon ground cinnamon

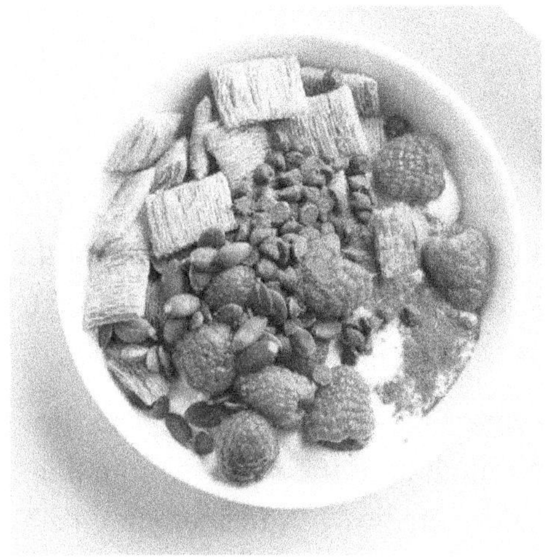

Directions

Spread yogurt in a bowl.

Add chocolate chips, raspberries, pumpkin seeds, cinnamon, and chopped wheat on top of the yogurt.

Nutrition Facts (per serving)

290	Calories
5g	Fat
48g	Carbs
18g	Protein

Rhubarb Oat Muffins

Prep Time: 20 mins   **Additional Time:** 25 mins   **Total Time:** 45 mins

Servings: 12   **Yield:** 12 servings

Ingredients

Nonstick cooking spray

1 ¾ cups regular rolled oats

¾ cup whole-wheat pastry flour or whole-wheat flour

½ cup all-purpose flour

½ cup packed brown sugar (see Tip)

1 teaspoon baking powder

½ teaspoon baking soda

¼ teaspoon salt

¾ cup buttermilk

½ cup refrigerated or frozen egg product, thawed, or 2 eggs, lightly beaten

2 tablespoons canola oil

1 teaspoon vanilla

1 cup finely chopped rhubarb

1 tablespoon packed brown sugar (see Tip)

½ teaspoon ground cinnamon

¼ cup chopped walnuts

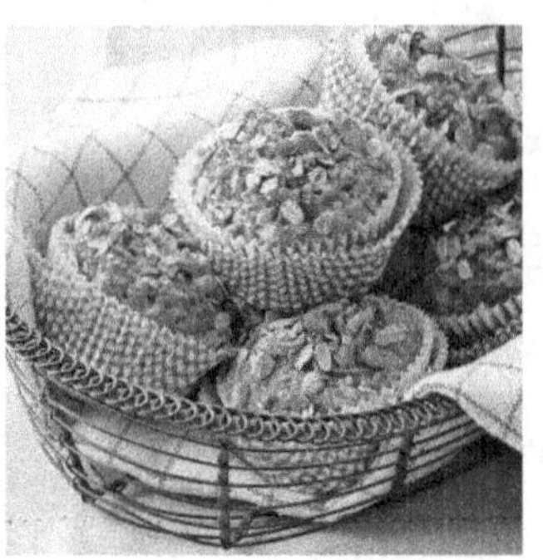

Directions

Warm the oven up to 350 degrees F. Paper bake cups should be used to line twelve 2 1/2-inch muffin pans. Spray cooking spray on the paper cups. Cooking spray can also be used to cover muffin cups.

Place 3/4 cup of the oats in a food processor. Cover it and run it until the oats are ground up. Put the food in a big bowl. Add another 3/4 cup of oats, the all-purpose flour, brown sugar, baking powder, baking soda, and salt. Also mix in the whole-wheat flour. Make a hole in the middle of the flour mix.

Mix the buttermilk, eggs, oil, and vanilla in a medium-sized bowl. Add the rhubarb and mix it in. All at once, add the rhubarb mixture to the flour mixture and stir just until the flour is wet. The batter should still have some lumps in it. Fill each muffin cup about three-quarters of the way to the top with the batter.

38

Mix brown sugar and cinnamon in a small bowl to make the crumb topping. Add the last 1/4 cup of oats and walnuts and mix them in. Put some on top of the muffin cup batter.

Bake for 20 to 22 minutes, or until a toothpick comes out clean. Place the muffin cups on a wire rack and let them cool for 5 minutes. Take out of the muffin tins.

Warm up and serve.

Tips

If you want to make the muffins without sugar, Splenda(R) Brown Sugar Blend is a good choice. To use 1/2 cup, follow the directions on the package.

How Healthy Is One Serving with a Substitute? The only difference is that it has 166 calories and 25 grams of carbs (6 grams of sugars).I don't think that a sugar replacement should be used in the streusel topping.

Nutrition Facts (per serving)

181	Calories
5g	Fat
30g	Carbs
5g	Protein

Apple Cinnamon Chia Pudding

Prep Time: 10 mins   **Additional Time:** 8 hrs   **Total Time:** 8 hrs 10 mins

Servings: 1   **Yield:** 1 cup

Ingredients

½ cup unsweetened almond milk or other nondairy milk

2 tablespoons chia seeds

2 teaspoons pure maple syrup

¼ teaspoon vanilla extract

¼ teaspoon ground cinnamon

½ cup diced apple, divided

1 tablespoon chopped toasted pecans, divided

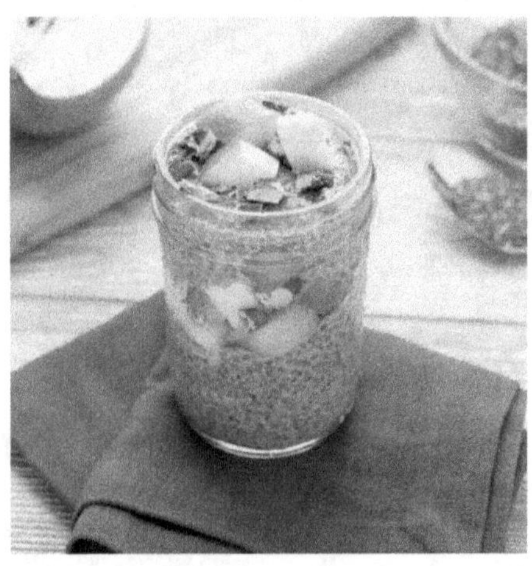

Directions

In a small bowl, mix almond milk, chia, maple syrup, vanilla, and cinnamon together. For at least eight hours or up to three days, cover and put in the fridge.

Mix well when you're ready to serve. Put about half of the pudding into a bowl or serving glass.

Then, put half of the apples and pecans on top. Put the rest of the pudding on top, then the apples and nuts.

Nutrition Facts (per serving)

233	Calories
13g	Fat
28g	Carbs
5g	Protein

Homemade Pizza Sauce

Cook Time: 30 mins   **Additional Time:** 2 hrs. 15 mins   **Total Time:** 2 hrs. 45 mins

Servings: 20   **Yield:** 5 cups

Ingredients

5 pounds cored whole tomatoes, fresh or frozen

3 tablespoons extra-virgin olive oil

2 medium onions, chopped

4 cloves garlic, minced

3/4 teaspoon dried basil or 1 tablespoon chopped fresh

3/4 teaspoon dried thyme or 1 tablespoon chopped fresh

3/4 teaspoon dried oregano or 1 tablespoon chopped fresh

1 ¾ teaspoons salt

½ teaspoon freshly ground pepper

1 to 2 teaspoons sugar (optional)

2 tablespoons tomato paste

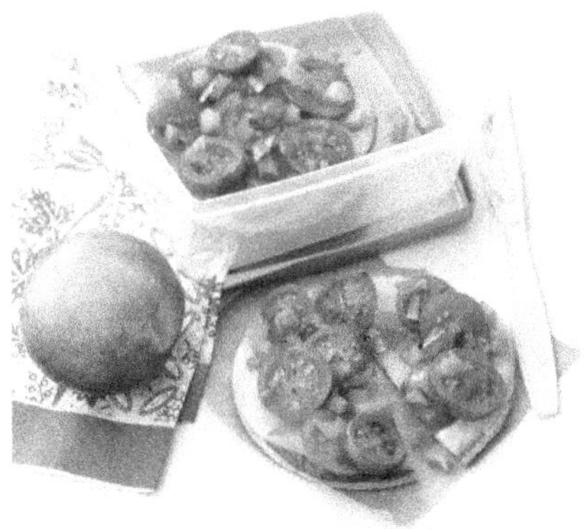

Directions

To prepare fresh tomatoes, boil a big saucepan of water. Make a tiny X in the bottom of each tomato and immerse in boiling water for 30 seconds to 2 minutes, or until the skins relax somewhat. Transfer to a dish of icy water for 1 minute. Peel using a paring knife, beginning at the X.

If using frozen tomatoes, run them under warm water and peel or wipe off the skin. Thaw in the fridge or the microwave until mostly thawed. Chop the tomatoes and save any liquid.

Preheat oil in a Dutch oven over medium heat. Stir in the onions and simmer for 4 to 6 minutes or until brown. Stir in the garlic and simmer for 1 minute.

Combine the tomatoes (with any liquid), basil, thyme, oregano, salt, pepper, and sugar (if using). Bring to a boil. Reduce the heat to a simmer and cook for approximately 2 hours or until the mixture is thick enough to resemble pizza sauce. Season to taste with extra salt, pepper, and/or sugar.

Transfer sauce to a blender, add tomato paste and mix until smooth. (Be cautious while puréeing hot liquids.)

Tips

Make Ahead Tip: Cover and refrigerate for up to three days, or freeze up to six months.

Nutrition Facts (per serving)

44	Calories
2g	Fat
5g	Carbs
1g	Protein

Muesli with Raspberries

Prep Time: 5 mins   **Total Time:** 5 mins

Servings: 1   **Yield:** about 1 3/4 cups

What is Muesli?

Muesli consists of rolled oats, nuts, seeds, and dried fruit. Muesli, unlike granola, is neither sweetened nor cooked with oil. Find your favorite brand from the store or create your own muesli.

Can I switch to plant-based milk?

Absolutely! We propose basic, unsweetened plant-based milk. Flavorings and sweeteners will alter both nutrition and taste.

Ingredients

⅓ cup muesli

1 cup raspberries

¾ cup low-fat milk

Directions

Top muesli with raspberries and serve with milk.

Nutrition Facts (per serving)

288	Calories
7g	Fat
52g	Carbs
13g	Protein

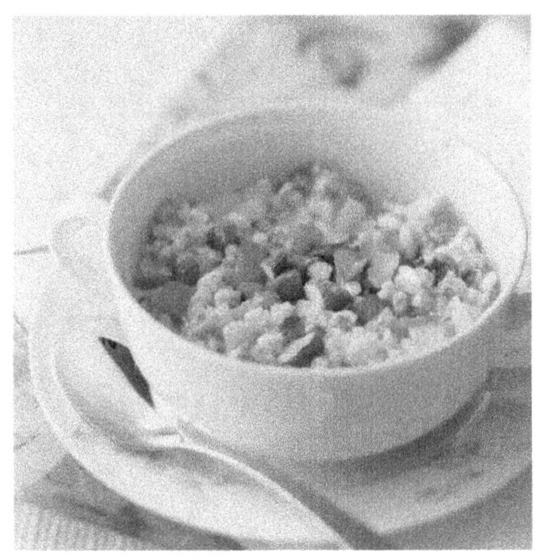

Almond-Matcha Green Smoothie Bowl

Prep Time: 15 mins   **Total Time:** 15 mins

Servings: 1   **Yield:** 1 bowl

Ingredients

½ cup snap or snow peas, trimmed

4 spears asparagus, tough ends removed, cut into 2-inch pieces

½ cup plain whole-milk yogurt

¼ cup chopped fresh dill

1 tablespoon lemon juice

1 tablespoon extra-virgin olive oil

1 clove garlic, minced

¼ teaspoon kosher salt

½ cup cooked farro

4 ounces baked tofu, cubed

3 radishes, sliced

1 tablespoon Toasted pumpkin seeds for garnish

Directions

Heat a medium saucepan of water to a boil. Cook for approximately 2 minutes, stirring in the snap (or snow) peas and asparagus until just soft. Rinse with cold water.

Combine yogurt, dill, lemon juice, oil, garlic, and salt in a small bowl.

Transfer farro to a shallow serving dish. Garnish with peas, asparagus, tofu, and radishes. Drizzle 2 tablespoons dressing over the top (keep the rest for later). Sprinkle with pumpkin seeds, if desired.

Nutrition Facts (per serving)

553	Calories
26g	Fat
56g	Carbs
29g	Protein

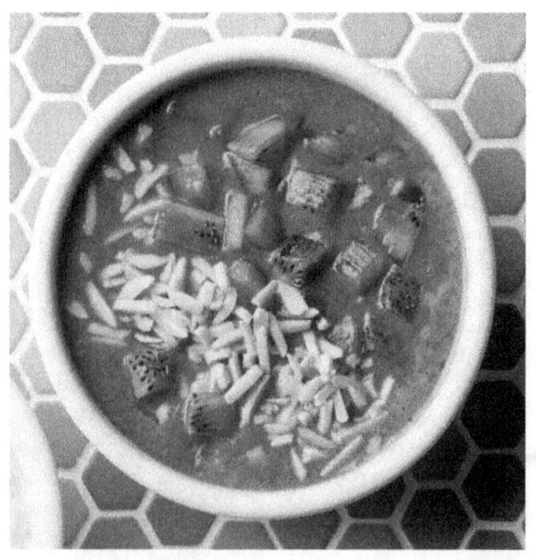

Peanut Butter Protein Overnight Oats

Prep Time: 5 mins   **Additional Time:** 7 hrs 55 mins   **Total Time:** 8 hrs

Servings: 1   **Yield:** 1 cups

Ingredients

½ cup soymilk or other plant-based milk

½ cup old-fashioned rolled oats (see Tip)

1 tablespoon pure maple syrup

1 tablespoon chia seeds

1 tablespoon powdered peanut butter

Pinch of salt

½ medium banana, sliced, or 1/2 cup berries

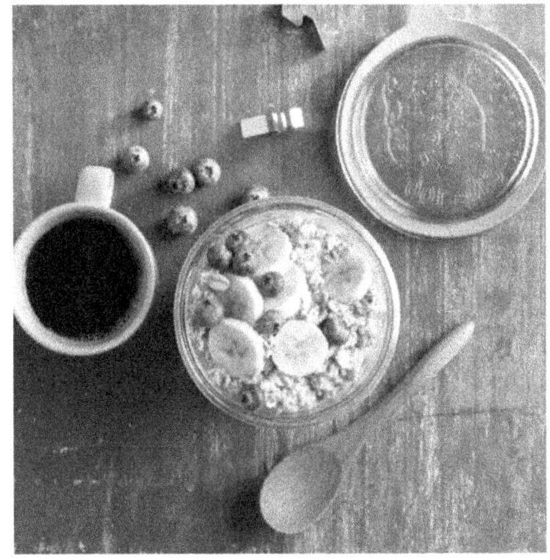

Directions

Combine soymilk (or other milk), oats, syrup, chia, powdered peanut butter, and salt in a 2-cup Mason jar. Refrigerate overnight.

Garnish with banana or berries.

Tips

People with celiac disease or gluten sensitivity should use "gluten-free" oats, since they are often cross-contaminated with wheat and barley.

To make ahead: Prepare through Step 1 and chill for up to four days.

Nutrition Facts (per serving)

368	Calories
9g	Fat
63g	Carbs
13g	Protein

POULTRY

Sheet-Pan Chicken Fajita Bowls

Prep Time: 20 mins   **Additional Time:** 20 mins   **Total Time:** 40 mins

Servings: 4   **Yield:** 4 servings

4 cups chopped stemmed kale

1 (15 ounce) can no-salt-added black beans, rinsed

¼ cup low-fat plain Greek yogurt

1 tablespoon lime juice

2 teaspoons water

Ingredients

2 teaspoons chili powder

2 teaspoons ground cumin

¾ teaspoon salt, divided

½ teaspoon garlic powder

½ teaspoon smoked paprika

¼ teaspoon ground pepper

2 tablespoons olive oil, divided

1 ¼ pounds chicken tenders

1 medium yellow onion, sliced

1 medium red bell pepper, sliced

1 medium green bell pepper, sliced

Directions

Preheat the oven to 425 degrees F and place a big rimmed baking sheet inside.

In a large bowl, combine chili powder, cumin, 1/2 tsp. salt, garlic powder, paprika, and ground pepper. Place 1 tsp of the spice mixture in a medium bowl and set aside. In a large bowl, whisk in 1 Tbsp. oil with the remaining spice combination. Toss in the chicken, onion, and red and green bell peppers until coated.

After removing the pan from the oven, treat it with cooking spray. Spread the chicken mixture evenly over the pan. Roast for fifteen minutes.

In a large dish, stir kale and black beans with remaining 1/4 tsp. salt and 1 Tbsp. olive oil.

Remove pan from oven. Stir together the chicken and veggies. Spread the greens and beans equally over the top. Roast for another 5 to 7 minutes, or until the chicken is fully cooked and the veggies are soft.

Combine yogurt, lime juice, and water with the reserved spice combination. Stir well.

Divide the chicken and vegetable mixture into four bowls. Drizzle with yogurt dressing and serve.

Tips

For simpler evening preparation, slice veggies the night before and chill.

To make ahead: Prepare the spice combination (Step 1) up to two days in advance; store in an airtight container.

Nutrition Facts (per serving)

343	Calories
10g	Fat
24g	Carbs
43g	Protein

Chicken Tagine

Servings: 8   **Yield:** 8 servings.

Ingredients

3 tablespoons extra-virgin olive oil

1 medium yellow onion, diced (about 1 cup)

Pinch of salt

1 tablespoon minced fresh ginger

4 garlic cloves, minced

2 teaspoons ground turmeric

1 teaspoon freshly ground black pepper

½ teaspoon ground cinnamon

½ preserved lemon peel, finely chopped

8 pitted Medjool dates, chopped

½ cup brown lentils

4 cups chicken stock

2 teaspoons kosher salt

1 pinch saffron

1 cup pitted olive oil

1 (15 ounce) can garbanzo beans, drained and rinsed

1 whole store-bought rotisserie chicken (3 to 4 pounds)

¼ cup chopped fresh flat-leaf parsley

Directions

Heat olive oil in a medium-high Dutch oven or heavy-bottomed pot with the onion and a touch of salt, and simmer for 2 minutes.

Cook for another minute after adding the ginger and garlic, then whisk in the turmeric, black pepper, and cinnamon for a further 30 seconds.

Mix in the preserved lemon, dates, and lentils. Pour in the stock, then add the salt and saffron. Bring to a boil, then lower to a simmer.

Add the olives and garbanzo beans. Cover the pan and heat for 25 minutes, turning periodically, until the lentils are cooked through.

Remove the chicken flesh from the skin and bones while cooking in the tagine.

Nutrition Facts (per serving)

710	Calories
20g	Fat
47g	Carbs
84g	Protein

Chipotle Chicken Quinoa Burrito Bowl

Active Time: 30 mins   **Total Time:** 30 mins

Servings: 4   **Yield:** 4 burrito bowls

Ingredients

1 tablespoon finely chopped chipotle peppers in adobo sauce

1 tablespoon extra-virgin olive oil

½ teaspoon garlic powder

½ teaspoon ground cumin

1 pound boneless, skinless chicken breast

¼ teaspoon salt

2 cups cooked quinoa

2 cups shredded romaine lettuce

1 cup canned pinto beans, rinsed

1 ripe avocado, diced

¼ cup prepared pico de gallo or other salsa

¼ cup shredded Cheddar or Monterey Jack cheese

Lime wedges for serving

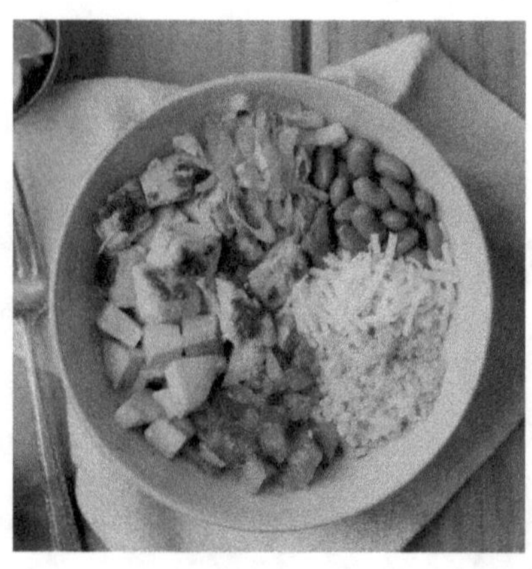

Directions

Preheat the grill or broiler to medium-high.

In a small dish, mix chipotles, oil, cumin, and garlic powder.

If broiling, oil a rimmed baking sheet or the grill rack (see Tip). Season the chicken with salt.

On the baking sheet that has been prepared, broil or grill the chicken for five or nine minutes.

After flipping, brush with the chipotle glaze, and cook for 3 to 5 minutes on the grill or 9 minutes under the broiler or until an instant-read thermometer inserted in the thickest section registers 165 degrees F.

Move to a sanitized chopping board. Dice into little pieces.

Fill each burrito bowl with the following ingredients: 1/2 cup quinoa, 1/2 cup chicken, 1/2 cup lettuce, 1/4 cup beans, 1/4 avocado, 1 tablespoon cheese, and 1 tablespoon pico de gallo (or other salsa).

Garnish with a wedge of lime.

Tips

To oil a grill rack, use tongs to hold a folded paper towel and rub it all over the rack. (Do not apply cooking spray to a hot grill.)

Nutrition Facts (per serving)

452	Calories
19g	Fat
36g	Carbs
36g	Protein

Slow-Cooker Chicken & White Bean Stew

Prep Time: 15 mins   **Active Time:** 10 min   **Additional Time:** 7 hrs. 20 mins

Total Time: 7 hrs. 45 mins   **Servings:** 6

Yield: 7 1/2 cups

Ingredients

1 pound dried cannellini beans, soaked overnight and drained (see Tip, above)

6 cups unsalted chicken broth

1 cup chopped yellow onion

1 cup sliced carrots

1 teaspoon finely chopped fresh rosemary

1 (4 ounce) Parmesan cheese rind plus 2/3 cup grated Parmesan, divided

2 bone-in chicken breasts (1 pound each)

4 cups chopped kale

1 tablespoon lemon juice

½ teaspoon kosher salt

½ teaspoon ground pepper

2 tablespoons extra-virgin olive oil

¼ cup flat-leaf parsley leaves

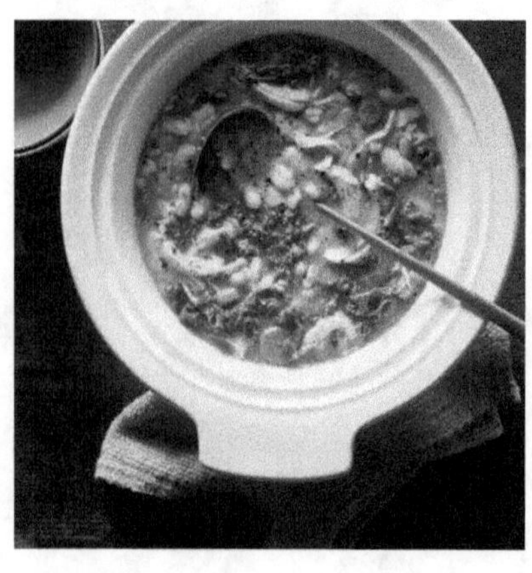

Directions

Combine the following ingredients in a 6-quart slow cooker: legumes, broth, onion, carrots, rosemary, and Parmesan rind. Add poultry on top. Cover and cook on low for 7 to 8 hours, or until the legumes and vegetables are fully cooked.

Transfer chicken to a clean chopping board and let cool for 10 minutes. Shred the chicken, discarding the bones.

Add greens to the slow cooker with the chicken. Cover and cook on high for 20 to 30 minutes, or until the kale is soft.

Add lemon juice, salt, and pepper; discard Parmesan rind. Serve the stew drizzled with oil and garnished with Parmesan and parsley.

Nutrition Facts (per serving)

493	Calories
11g	Fat
54g	Carbs
44g	Protein

Broccoli, Chicken Sausage & Orzo Skillet

Prep Time: 20 mins   **Additional Time:** 10 mins   **Total Time:** 30 mins

Servings: 4   **Yield**: 4 servings

Ingredients

2 teaspoons olive oil

6 ounces cooked chicken sausage, such as Al Fresco Sweet Italian, cut into 1/4-inch slices

½ cup chopped onion

1 cup whole-wheat orzo

3 cloves garlic, minced

2 ½ cups low-sodium chicken broth

¼ teaspoon crushed red pepper, plus more for garnish

¼ teaspoon kosher salt

1 pound broccoli, trimmed, or 4 cups broccoli florets

¼ cup grated Parmesan cheese, plus more for garnish

2 teaspoons lemon zest

Directions

Heat oil in a 12-inch cast-iron or heavy skillet on medium-high heat. Cook, tossing occasionally, until sausage is browned, about 3 to 4 minutes. Cook for a further minute, tossing in the orzo and garlic.

Add broth, crushed red pepper, and salt. Bring to a boil. Stir in the broccoli (or broccoli). Reduce the heat, cover, and let the orzo simmer for 8 to 10 minutes or until tender. Uncover and continue cooking until the broth has been absorbed.

Stir in the Parmesan and lemon zest. If preferred, sprinkle with extra Parmesan and crushed red pepper before serving.

Nutrition Facts (per serving)

333	Calories
10g	Fat
42g	Carbs
18g	Protein

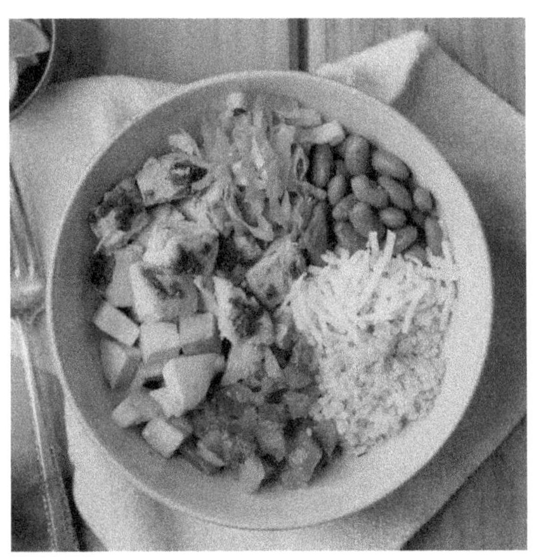

Lemon-Tahini Couscous with Chicken & Vegetables

Active Time: 25 mins   **Total Time:** 25 mins

Servings: 4   **Yield:** 6 cups

Ingredients

1 cup whole-wheat pearl couscous (see Tip)

¼ cup tahini

¼ cup water

2 teaspoons lemon zest

2 tablespoons lemon juice

2 tablespoons olive oil, divided

½ teaspoon salt

¼ teaspoon ground pepper

¼ teaspoon crushed red pepper

1 clove garlic, minced

2 cups sliced mushrooms (half of a 10-oz. package)

½ medium red bell pepper, chopped

4 cups coleslaw mix (half of a 12- to 14-oz. package)

4 cups baby spinach (half of a 5-oz. bag)

12 ounces cooked chicken breast, chopped (about 2 1/2 cups)

¼ cup toasted sliced almonds

¼ cup crumbled reduced-fat feta cheese

1 tablespoon chopped fresh parsley

1 lemon, cut into wedges (Optional)

Directions

Cook couscous in a medium saucepan per package instructions. Fluff with a fork, then set aside.

Combine tahini, water, lemon juice, and 1 Tbsp oil, salt, pepper, and crushed red pepper in a small bowl. Whisk well and leave away.

Heat the remaining 1 Tbsp. oil over medium-high heat in a large nonstick skillet. Cook for about 30 seconds or until the garlic becomes aromatic. Cook for about 3 minutes, stirring in the mushrooms and bell pepper to release their juice.

Add coleslaw mix and spinach, stirring until wilted (approximately 2 minutes). Cook for 2 to 4 minutes, stirring in the chicken, couscous, and tahini sauce until thoroughly cooked.

Add almonds, feta, parsley, and lemon zest. If desired, serve with lemon slices.

Nutrition Facts (per serving)

528	Calories
23g	Fat
42g	Carbs
40g	Protein

Chicken Tinga Tostadas

Active Time: 15 mins   **Total Time:** 25 min   **Servings:** 4

Ingredients

8 corn tortillas

Cooking spray

2 ⅔ cups Chicken Tinga

1 (15 ounce) can low-sodium refried beans

½ cup crumbled cheese

½ cup chopped fresh cilantro

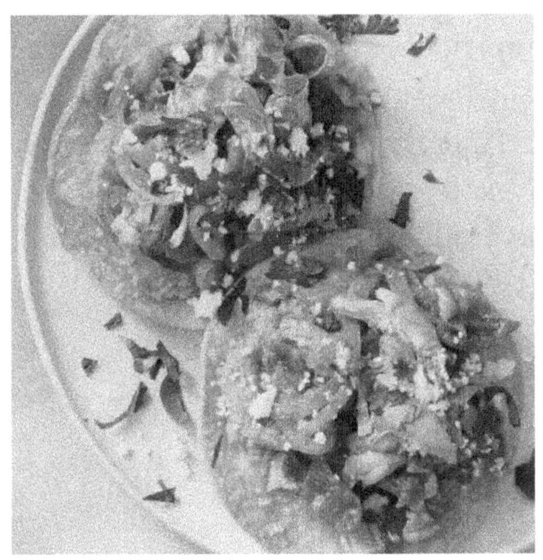

Directions

Preheat the oven to 350°F.

Place tortillas on a baking sheet in a single layer and brush both sides with cooking spray. Bake for approximately 12 minutes, flipping once, until crispy.

Heat chicken tinga and refried beans in separate pots until steamed. Divide the beans evenly among the tortillas, then top with 1/3 cup chicken and 1 tablespoon each cheese and cilantro.

Nutrition Facts (per serving)

345	Calories
10g	Fat
44g	Carbs
21g	Protein

One-Pot Spinach, Chicken Sausage & Feta Pasta

Active Time: 20 mins   **Total Time:** 20 mins

Servings: 4   **Yield:** 4 servings

Ingredients

2 tablespoons olive oil

3 links cooked chicken sausage (9 ounces), sliced into rounds

1 cup diced onion (see Tip)

1 clove garlic, minced

1 (8 ounce) can no-salt-added tomato sauce

4 cups lightly packed baby spinach (half of a 5-ounce box)

6 cups cooked whole-wheat rotini pasta

¼ cup chopped pitted Kalamata olives

½ cup finely crumbled feta cheese

¼ cup chopped fresh basil (Optional)

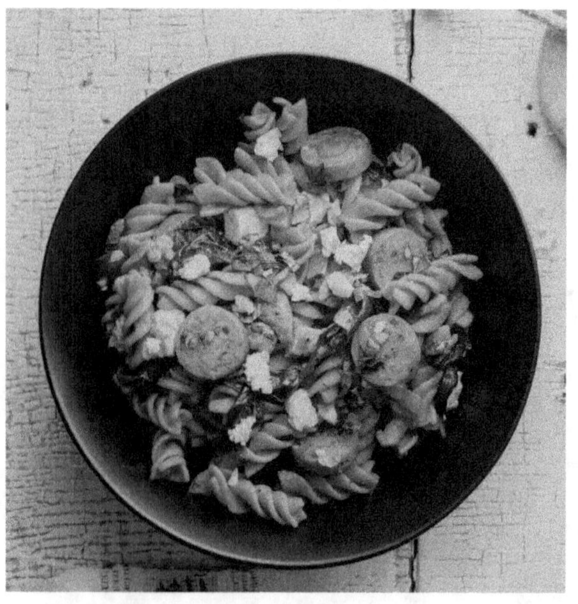

Directions

Heat oil in a big, straight-sided skillet over medium-high heat. Cook, stirring constantly, until the onion begins to brown, about 4 to 6 minutes.

Cook, stirring frequently, until the tomato sauce is boiling and the spinach has wilted, about 3 to 5 minutes. To prevent the pasta from sticking, add 1 to 2 teaspoons of water. If using, stir in the feta and basil.

Nutrition Facts (per serving)

487	Calories
20g	Fat
59g	Carbs
23g	Protein

Chicken & Vegetable Penne with Parsley-Walnut Pesto

Prep Time: 20 mins   **Additional Time:** 10 mins   **Total Time**: 30 mins

Servings: 4   **Yield:** 8 cups

Ingredients

¾ cup chopped walnuts

1 cup lightly packed parsley leaves

2 cloves garlic, crushed and peeled

½ teaspoon plus 1/8 teaspoon salt

⅛ teaspoon ground pepper

2 tablespoons olive oil

⅓ cup grated Parmesan cheese

1 ½ cups shredded or sliced cooked skinless chicken breast (8 oz.)

6 ounces whole-wheat penne or fusilli pasta (1 3/4 cups)

8 ounces green beans, trimmed and halved crosswise (2 cups)

2 cups cauliflower florets (8 oz.)

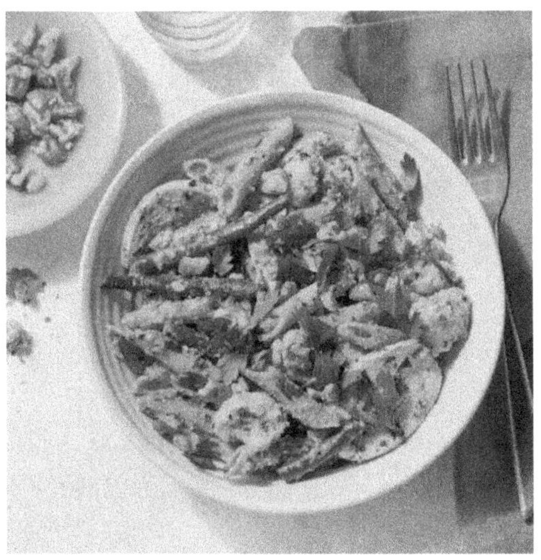

Directions

Bring a large saucepan of water to a boil.

Place the walnuts in a small bowl and microwave on high for 2 to 2 1/2 minutes, or until they are gently toasted and aromatic. (Alternatively, toast the walnuts in a small, dry skillet over medium-low heat, stirring frequently, until they are aromatic, which should take approximately 2 to 3 minutes.

Transfer to a plate and allow to cool. Reserve 1/4 cup for toppings.

In a food processor, combine the remaining half-cup of walnuts, parsley, garlic, salt, and pepper. Grind the nuts until they are finely ground. While the motor is in operation, gradually introduce oil through the feed tube. Pulse the Parmesan until it is fully incorporated. The pesto should be scraped into a large basin. Chicken should be incorporated.

In the interim, cook the pasta in boiling water for four minutes. Cover and simmer until the pasta is al dente (nearly mushy) and the vegetables are cooked, about 5 to 7 minutes.

Before draining, remove 3/4 cup of the cooking water and swirl it into the pesto-chicken combination to reheat it up slightly.

Drain the pasta and vegetables and combine with the pesto-chicken mixture. Toss to saturate evenly.

Divide among four pasta dishes, then top each with 1 tablespoon of the saved walnuts.

Nutrition Facts (per serving)

514	Calories
27g	Fat
43g	Carbs
31g	Protein

Slow-Cooker Chicken & Chickpea Soup

Prep Time: 20 mins   **Additional Time:** 4 hrs   **Total Time:** 4 hrs 20 mins

Servings: 6   **Yield:** 12 cups

Ingredients

1 ½ cups dried chickpeas, soaked overnight

4 cups water

1 large yellow onion, finely chopped

1 (15 ounce) can no-salt-added diced tomatoes, preferably fire-roasted

2 tablespoons tomato paste

4 cloves garlic, finely chopped

1 bay leaf

4 teaspoons ground cumin

4 teaspoons paprika

¼ teaspoon cayenne pepper

¼ teaspoon ground pepper

2 pounds bone-in chicken thighs, skin removed, trimmed

1 (14 ounce) can artichoke hearts, drained and quartered

¼ cup halved pitted oil-cured olives

½ teaspoon salt

¼ cup chopped fresh parsley or cilantro

Directions

Transfer the chickpeas to a 6-quart or larger slow cooker after draining them. The water should be stirred with onion, tomato liquid, tomato paste, garlic, bay leaf, cumin, paprika, cayenne, and pepper. Include. Cover the pot and cook on low for 8 hours or on high for 4 hours.

Transfer the chicken to a clean slicing board and allow it to cool slightly. The bay leaf should be discarded. Combine the artichokes, olives, and salt in the slow cooker.

Discard the bones after shredding the poultry. Incorporate the poultry into the soup. Garnish with cilantro or parsley.

Tips

To make ahead: Refrigerate for three days or freeze for three months.

Nutrition Facts (per serving)

447	Calories
15g	Fat
43g	Carbs
34g	Protein

Ancho Chicken Breast with Black Beans, Bell Peppers & Scallions

Prep Time: 45 mins   **Total Time:** 45 mins

Servings: 4   **Yield:** 4 servings

Ingredients

Beans

1 tablespoon extra-virgin olive oil

3 cloves garlic, minced

1 teaspoon cumin seeds

2 (15 ounce) cans low-sodium black beans, rinsed

Juice of 1 lime

¼ teaspoon kosher salt

Chicken & Vegetables

16 scallions, trimmed

3 medium red bell peppers, cut into 1-inch strips

1 ½ tablespoons extra-virgin olive oil plus 2 teaspoons, divided

¾ teaspoon kosher salt, divided

¼ teaspoon ground pepper

2 (8 ounce) boneless, skinless chicken breasts, trimmed and halved crosswise

1 teaspoon ancho chile powder (see Tips)

½ teaspoon ground cinnamon

½ teaspoon unsweetened cocoa powder

1 teaspoon brown sugar

Directions

To prepare the beans: In a medium saucepan, heat 1 tablespoon of oil over medium heat. Stir in the garlic and cumin seeds and simmer for 30 seconds to 1 minute, until aromatic and beginning to brown.

Cook until heated, stirring in the beans, lime juice, and 1/4 teaspoon salt, for 2 to 4 minutes. Remove from the heat and mash with a potato masher until nearly smooth.

Refrigerate 1/2 cup of mashed beans for later use (see Tips below). Cover the leftover beans to keep them heated.

To make chicken and vegetables: Position the rack in the upper third of the oven and preheat the broiler to high. Line a rimmed baking sheet with foil.

In a large bowl, combine scallions and bell peppers with 1 1/2 teaspoons oil and 1/4 teaspoon salt and pepper.

Transfer to the prepared baking sheet. Broil the vegetables, tossing twice, for 8 to 12 minutes, or until blackened.

Meanwhile, put the chicken between two large pieces of plastic wrap. Using the smooth side of a meat mallet or a heavy saucepan, pound to an equal thickness of 1/2 inch.

In a small bowl, combine the chile powder, cinnamon, cocoa, brown sugar, and remaining 1/2 teaspoon salt. Brush the remaining 2 teaspoons of oil onto both sides of the chicken, then coat with the spice mixture.

Coat a big grill pan or skillet with cooking spray and set it over medium-high heat. Reduce the heat to medium, and add half of the chicken.

Cook for 2 to 4 minutes per side, or until an instant-read thermometer inserted in the thickest section reaches 165 degrees Fahrenheit.

Repeat with the remaining chicken, lowering the heat as needed.

Place 2/3 cup beans on four dinner plates, then top with scallions, bell peppers, and chicken.

Tips

Ancho chiles- dried poblano peppers, are one of the most popular dried chiles in Mexico. Ancho Chile powder has a mild, sweet, spicy flavor. Look for it among the exotic spices at large supermarkets or Mexican grocers.

Make black bean tacos with leftovers for lunch. Spread 1/2 cup of leftover beans on two corn tortillas. Top each taco with 1/4 cup chopped romaine lettuce and tomato, 1 tablespoon each of shredded Cheddar cheese and tomato salsa, and a squeeze of lime juice.

Nutrition Facts (per serving)

396	Calories
14g	Fat
36g	Carbs
32g	Protein

Slow-Cooker Chicken & Orzo with Tomatoes & Olives

Active Time: 15 mins   **Total Time:** 2 hrs 15 mins

Servings: 4   **Yield:** 4 servings

Ingredients

1 pound boneless, skinless chicken breasts, trimmed

1 cup low-sodium chicken broth

2 medium tomatoes, chopped

1 medium onion, halved and sliced

Zest and juice of 1 lemon

1 teaspoon herbes de Provence

½ teaspoon salt

½ teaspoon ground pepper

¾ cup whole-wheat orzo

⅓ cup quartered black or green olives

2 tablespoons chopped fresh parsley

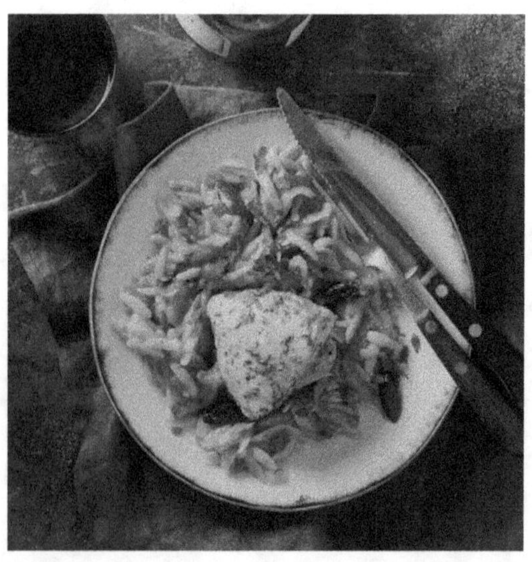

Directions

Cut each chicken breast half into four pieces. In a 6-quart slow cooker, combine the chicken, broth, tomatoes, onion, lemon zest, lemon juice, herbes de Provence, and salt and pepper.

Cook for one hour and 30 minutes on high or three hours and 30 minutes on low. Stir in the orzo and olives; cover and cook until the orzo is cooked, about 30 minutes longer.

Allow to cool slightly. Sprinkle with parsley before serving.

Nutrition Facts (per serving)

278	Calories
5g	Fat
30g	Carbs
29g	Protein

Chicken & Cucumber Lettuce Wraps with Peanut Sauce

Prep Time: 40 mins   **Total Time:** 40 mins

Servings: 4   **Yield:** 8 lettuce wraps

Ingredients

¼ cup creamy peanut butter

2 tablespoons low-sodium soy sauce

2 tablespoons honey

2 tablespoons water

2 teaspoons toasted sesame oil

2 teaspoons olive oil

3 scallions, sliced, white and green parts separated

1 serrano pepper, seeded and minced (2 tsp.)

1 tablespoon minced fresh ginger

2 teaspoons minced fresh garlic

1 pound ground chicken breast

1 cup diced jicama

16 Bibb lettuce leaves

1 cup cooked brown rice

1 cup halved and thinly sliced English cucumber

½ cup fresh cilantro leaves

Lime wedges, for serving

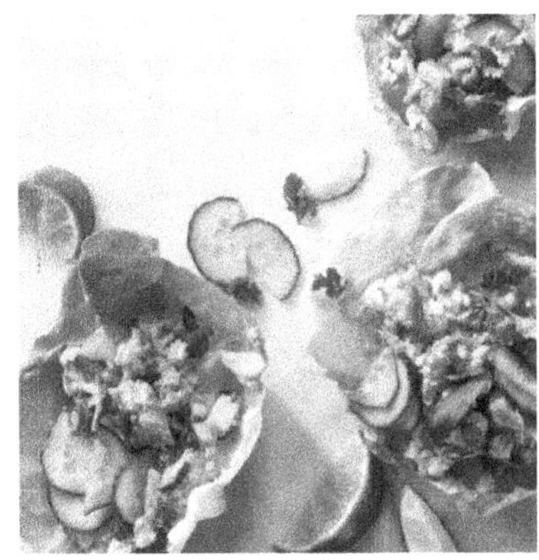

Directions

Combine peanut butter, soy sauce, honey, water, and sesame oil in a small mixing basin.

In a large nonstick skillet, heat olive oil over medium heat. Add the scallion whites, serrano, ginger, and garlic; simmer for about 2 minutes, or until softened.

Cook, breaking up the chicken with a spoon or potato masher, until it is cooked through, about 3 to 4 minutes.

Add the peanut sauce to the chicken mixture and heat for 3 minutes, or until thickened. Remove from heat. Stir in the jicama and scallion greens.

To serve, arrange 8 stacks of two lettuce leaves each. Divide the rice, chicken, cucumber, and cilantro among the lettuce cups. Serve with lime wedges.

Tips

Serves 4: 2 lettuce wraps each

Nutrition Facts (per serving)

521	Calories
26g	Fat
44g	Carbs
34g	Protein

Slow-Cooker Chicken with Rosemary & Mushrooms over Linguine

Prep Time: 20 mins   **Additional Time:** 4 hrs 5 mins   **Total Time:** 4 hrs 25 mins

Servings: 4   **Yield:** 4 servings

Ingredients

1 cup unsalted chicken stock

2 ½ tablespoons all-purpose flour

1 cup sliced shallots (from 4 shallots)

8 ounces sliced fresh cremini mushrooms

4 ounces sliced fresh shiitake mushrooms

⅓ cup dry Marsala wine

2 teaspoons chopped fresh rosemary

8 boneless, skinless chicken thighs (about 1 1/2 pounds)

¾ teaspoon kosher salt

½ teaspoon black pepper

8 ounces uncooked whole-wheat linguine

2 tablespoons whole fresh flat-leaf parsley leaves

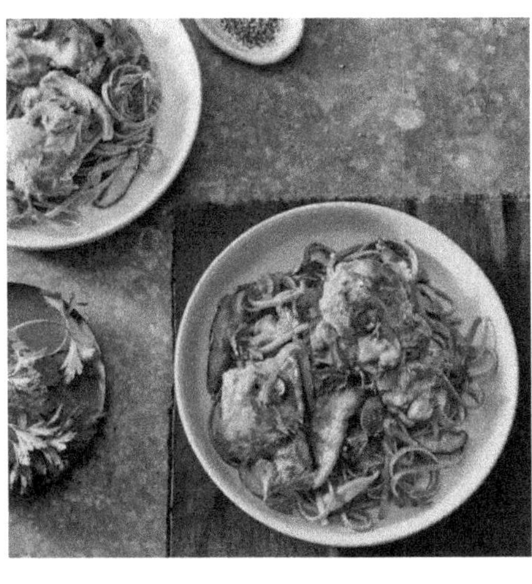

Directions

Whisk the stock and flour in a 5- to 6-quart slow cooker until they are thoroughly combined. Place the rosemary, Marsala, shallots, and mushrooms in the slow cooker.

Place the chicken in the slow cooker, ensconced among the vegetables and liquid, and season it with salt and pepper.

Cover the dish and cook on low for four hours, or until the chicken is fully cooked and the sauce has thickened.

Transfer the chicken from the slow cooker to a serving platter, reserving the simmering liquid and vegetables in the cooker.

Transfer the simmering liquid and vegetables to a 2-quart saucepan and heat over medium-high until boiling.

Cook the sauce, stirring intermittently, until it is reduced to 2 cups, which should take approximately 5 minutes.

Linguine should be cooked in accordance with the instructions on the container, excluding the salt and fat. The pasta should be drained.

Distribute the linguine equitably among four bowls and add the chicken on top. Apply the marinade on top. Distribute the parsley uniformly.

Tips

Multicooker Directions: In Step 1, whisk together the stock and flour in the inner pot of a 6-quart multicooker until well combined; then add the shallots, mushrooms, Marsala, and rosemary. Sprinkle the chicken with salt and pepper, then place it in the saucepan, nestled among the vegetables and liquid. Lock the lid and turn the pressure valve to "Venting." Cook on SLOW COOK [Normal] for approximately 4 hours, or until the chicken is cooked and the sauce has thickened. Turn off the cooker. In Step 2, move the chicken to a serving tray while keeping the cooking liquid and vegetables in the saucepan. With the lid removed, press SAUTÉ [Normal]. Bring to a boil and simmer uncovered, stirring frequently, until the sauce has reduced to 2 cups. Complete Step 3.

Nutrition Facts (per serving)

463	Calories
9g	Fat
53g	Carbs
49g	Protein

Chicken & Sun-Dried Tomato Orzo

Cook Time: 30 mins   **Total Time:** 30 mins

Servings: 4

Yield: 12 to 4 oz. chicken & cups pasta

Ingredients

8 ounces of orzo, preferably whole-wheat

One cup of water

Chopped sun-dried tomatoes, approximately half a cup (not oil-packed), divided

1 diced plum tomato

1 peeled garlic clove

3 teaspoons of minced fresh marjoram, divided

1 tablespoon of red wine vinegar

4 boneless, skinless chicken breasts, trimmed (1-1 1/4 pounds)

 2 teaspoons plus

1 tablespoon extra-virgin olive oil, divided

1/2 teaspoon of salt

1/2 teaspoon of freshly ground pepper

1 9-ounce package of frozen artichoke hearts, thawed

½ cup of finely shredded Romano cheese, divided

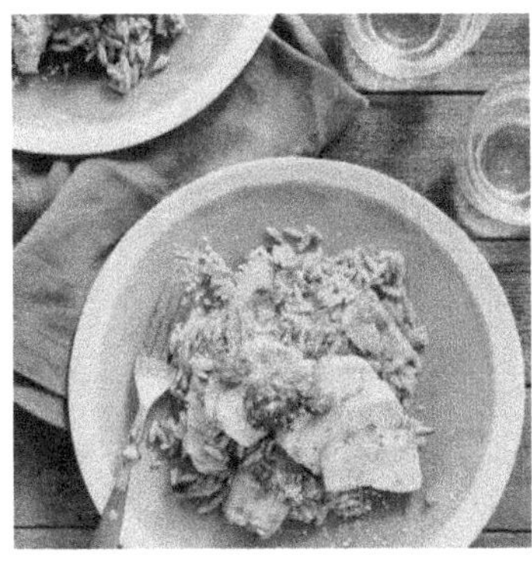

Directions

Follow the instructions on the package to cook orzo in a large saucepan of boiling water for 8 to 10 minutes or until it is just tender. Rinse and drain.

In the interim, blend 1 cup of water, 1/4 cup of sun-dried tomatoes, a plum tomato, garlic, 2 teaspoons of marjoram, 2 teaspoons of vinegar, and 2 teaspoons of oil in a blender. Blend until only a few crumbs remain.

Sprinkle salt and pepper over the chicken on both sides. Heat the remaining 1 tablespoon of oil in a large skillet over medium-high heat.

Cook the chicken for 3 to 5 minutes on each side, regulating the heat as necessary to prevent scorching. Transfer the dish to a platter and cover it with foil to maintain its temperature.

Add the tomato sauce to the pan and bring it to a simmer. Add 1/2 cup of sauce to a small basin. Combine the orzo, artichoke centers, and 6 tablespoons of cheese in the pan with the remaining 1/4 cup of sun-dried tomatoes.

Stir the mixture until it is fully heated, which should take approximately one to two minutes. Distribute among four dishes.

Cut the chicken into thin slices. Top each serving of pasta with sliced chicken, 2 tablespoons of the conserved tomato sauce, and a sprinkle of the remaining cheese and marjoram.

Nutrition Facts (per serving)

456	Calories
12g	Fat
54g	Carbs
36g	Protein

MEAT 15

Stuffed Zucchini Andalouse (Zucchini Ham Beef)

Prep: 15 min   **Cook Time:** 30 min   **Ready:** 45 min

Servings: 6

Ingredients

6 small zucchini

2 tablespoons onions chopped

3 tablespoons mushrooms chopped

3 tablespoons green bell peppers chopped

⅓ Cup tomatoes chopped

¼ cup ham cooked, chopped

½ teaspoon garlic minced

½ cup beef cooked, chopped

1 ⅓ cups bread crumbs soft, lightly piled

½ clove garlic chopped

2 tablespoons stock

⅛ Teaspoon salt

⅛ Teaspoon black pepper

Directions

Cook zucchini for 5 minutes in salted water; cut lengthwise to remove pulp.

Mix the pulp with remaining ingredients; fill zucchini to bursting and bake for 30 minutes at 350 degrees Fahrenheit.

Nutrition Facts

Serving Size 168g (5.9oz)

Amount per Serving

Calories 119	Fat 2g
Cholesterol 0mg	Sodium 253mg
Carbohydrate 7g	Fiber 3g

Sugars g   Protein 10g

Spicy Red Curry Beef & Rice

Active Time: 20 mins   **Total Time:** 20 mins

Servings: 4

Ingredients

1 (13.5-ounce) can light coconut milk

4 teaspoons red curry paste

2 teaspoons dark brown sugar

2 teaspoons fish sauce

¼ teaspoon crushed red pepper

1 ½ cups sliced red bell pepper

1 cup sliced onion

12 ounces beef tenderloin, thinly sliced

1 cup torn fresh basil leaves

2 tablespoons fresh lime juice

½ teaspoon kosher salt

2 cups hot cooked brown basmati rice

4 lime wedges

Directions

Pour coconut cream (thick layer on top of can) into a large skillet and mix in curry paste. Bring to a boil over medium high heat. Bring to a boil.

Add the remaining coconut milk, sugar, fish sauce, and red pepper. Cook for 2 minutes, stirring constantly.

Add the bell pepper and onion, then reduce the heat to medium and simmer for 4 minutes.

Cook for 3 minutes, tossing regularly, until the steak is cooked through.

Remove the skillet from the heat and mix in the basil, lime juice, and salt. Serve the meat combination with rice and lime wedges.

Nutrition Facts (per serving)

334	Calories
11g	Fat
36g	Carbs
24g	Protein

Ground Beef & Potatoes Skillet

Active Time: 40 mins   **Total Time:** 40 mins

Servings: 6

Ingredients

3 tablespoons extra-virgin olive oil, divided

1 pound 90% lean ground beef

2 teaspoons ground cumin

¾ teaspoon salt

¼ teaspoon ground pepper

3 medium Yukon Gold potatoes, diced (1/2-inch)

1 medium yellow onion, chopped

1 yellow bell pepper, diced (1/2-inch)

1 poblano pepper, diced (1/2-inch)

2 cloves garlic, minced

1 bunch lacinato kale, stemmed and roughly chopped

2 plum tomatoes, cored and diced (1/2-inch)

1 scallion, thinly sliced crosswise (optional)

Directions

Warm 1 tablespoon oil in a large skillet over medium-high heat. Cook, tossing frequently to break up the meat, until uniformly browned, about 6 minutes. Transfer the meat to a paper-towel-lined dish; do not clean the pan.

Add 1 tablespoon oil to the pan's drippings. Cook, stirring periodically, until potatoes begin to caramelize and become soft, about 20 minutes. Add the potatoes to the platter with the beef.

Heat the remaining 1 tablespoon oil in the skillet over medium heat. Cook until the onion, bell pepper, and poblano are soft, about 6 minutes, stirring occasionally. Cook, stirring frequently, for about 1 minute, or until garlic is fragrant.

Cook, tossing frequently, until the kale wilts and the tomatoes are heated through about 3 minutes. Add in the steak and potatoes. Sprinkle with sliced onions, if desired

Nutrition Facts (per serving)

322	Calories
15g	Fat
30g	Carbs
20g	Protein

Cheesy Ground Beef & Cauliflower Casserole

Active Time: 30 mins   **Total Time:** 30 mins

Servings: 6

Ingredients

1 tablespoon extra-virgin olive oil

½ cup chopped onion

1 medium green bell pepper, chopped

1 pound lean ground beef

3 cups bite-size cauliflower florets

3 cloves garlic, minced

2 tablespoons chili powder

2 teaspoons ground cumin

1 teaspoon dried oregano

½ teaspoon salt

¼ teaspoon ground chipotle

1 (15 ounce) can no-salt-added petite-diced tomatoes

2 cups shredded extra-sharp Cheddar cheese

⅓ cup sliced pickled jalapeños

Directions

Position the rack in the upper third of the oven. Preheat the broiler to high.

Heat the oil in a large broiler-safe skillet over medium heat. Stir in the onion and bell pepper and simmer for about 5 minutes or until softened.

Cook, tossing and breaking up the beef into smaller pieces, until no longer pink, about 5 to 7 minutes.

Add garlic, chili powder, cumin, oregano, salt, and chipotle; simmer for 1 minute or until fragrant.

Add the tomatoes and juices; bring to a simmer and cook, stirring periodically, until the liquid has been reduced and the cauliflower is cooked, about 3 minutes more. Remove from heat.

Top the meat mixture with cheese and jalapeño slices. Broil for 2 to 3 minutes or until the cheese has melted and browned in spots.

Nutrition Facts (per serving)

351	Calories
23g	Fat
11g	Carbs
26g	Protein

Italian-Style Beef & Pork Meatballs

Active Time: 20 mins   **Total Time:** 35 mins

Ingredients

3 large eggs, lightly beaten

1 cup finely chopped onion

¾ cup panko breadcrumbs, preferably whole-wheat

¾ cup chopped fresh parsley

½ cup grated Parmesan cheese

3 large cloves garlic, minced

1 tablespoon Italian seasoning

1 ½ teaspoons salt

1 teaspoon ground pepper

1 ½ pounds lean ground beef

1 ½ pounds ground pork

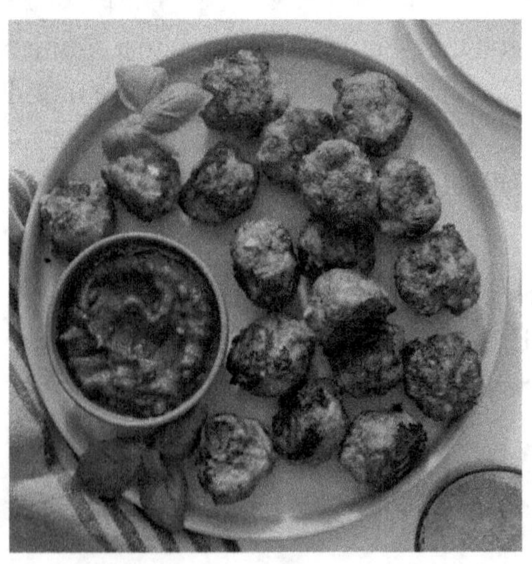

Directions

Place racks in the upper and bottom thirds of the oven and warm to 450°F. Line two large, rimmed baking pans with foil and coat with cooking spray.

In a large bowl, combine the eggs, onion, panko, parsley, parmesan, garlic, Italian seasoning, salt, and pepper.

Combine beef and pork. Mix lightly with your hands until just blended (don't overmix).

Shape 48 meatballs using a generous 2 teaspoons each. Place one inch apart on the prepared baking pans.

Bake the meatballs for approximately 15 minutes, or until an instant-read thermometer inserted in the center reads 165°F.

Tip

Try these meatballs in one of these easy dinner recipes.

To prepare Meatball Pesto & Gnocchi Bake, cook 1 lb. gnocchi in 1 Tbsp. olive oil in a large broiler-safe skillet over medium heat until browned, about 5 minutes. Stir in 18 meatballs and 1/3 cup pesto, ricotta, and water until evenly coated. Spread the mixture evenly, then top with 1/4 cup grated Parmesan cheese and 3 tablespoons breadcrumbs. Broil on high for 1 to 2 minutes, or until golden brown. (Serves 6)

To make Meatball Stuffed Shells, cook 18 large pasta shells. In a mixing dish, combine 1 cup ricotta, 1/4 cup grated Parmesan cheese, one big egg, and a sprinkling of salt and pepper. Place 1 cup marinara sauce in a 9-by-13-inch baking dish. Stuff each shell with one meatball and 1 tablespoon of the ricotta mixture; place in the baking dish, open side up. Top with 1 cup sauce and 1/4 cup Parmesan. Cover with foil. Bake at 375°F for 30 minutes or until the sauce is bubbling. Uncover and bake for another 10 minutes.

To prepare the Meatballs over Cheesy Polenta (serves 6), bring 4 cups of water to a boil in a medium saucepan over high heat. Slowly mix in 1 cup of cornmeal and decrease the heat to a simmer. Cook, stirring periodically, until the polenta is thick and soft, about 20 minutes. Remove from heat. Combine 1 1/4 cups shredded sharp Cheddar cheese, 4 sliced scallions, 1 Tbsp butter, and 1/4 tsp salt and pepper. Serve 16 heated meatballs over polenta. (Serves four)

Nutrition Facts (per serving)

216	Calories
10g	Fat
6g	Carbs
26g	Protein

Slow-Cooker Balsamic Short Ribs

Active Time: 30 mins   **Additional Time:** 4 hrs   **Total Time:** 4 hrs 30 mins

Servings: 6   **Yield:** 6 servings

Ingredients

6 bone-in beef short ribs (about 3 1/4 pounds)

¾ teaspoon salt, divided

½ teaspoon ground pepper

2 tablespoons extra-virgin olive oil, divided

1 medium onion, sliced

2 tablespoons tomato paste

2 cloves garlic, chopped

1 teaspoon chopped fresh thyme

1 cup balsamic vinegar

½ cup low-sodium beef broth

2 tablespoons cornstarch

¼ cup water

1 tablespoon Chopped fresh parsley

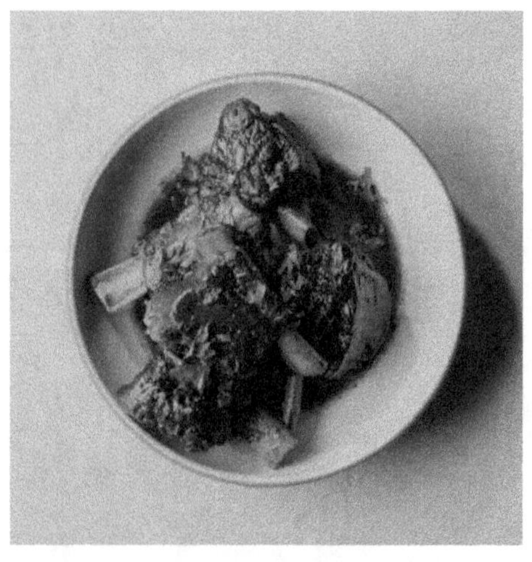

Directions

Sprinkle the ribs with 1/2 teaspoon of salt and pepper. Place a large skillet over medium-high heat and heat 1 tablespoon of oil. The ribs should be cooked until they are golden brown on all sides, which should take approximately five minutes.

Transfer the mixture to a slow cooker that is at least six quarts in capacity.

Cook the onion for 3 to 5 minutes, stirring frequently, until it begins to caramelize. Stir in the garlic, thyme, and tomato paste, and allow the mixture to simmer for one minute while whisking.

Scrape away any browned parts and add the vinegar, allowing it to simmer for 3 to 5 minutes. The broth should be added to the slow cooker after the transfer. Cover and cook on high for 4 hours or on low for 8 hours.

Transfer the ribs to a serving plate. Transfer the liquid to a medium saucepan and raise it to a boil over high heat. Whisk the cornstarch and water in a small dish, and then add it to the simmering liquid.

Cook the mixture, whisking continuously, until it thickens, which should take approximately two minutes. Incorporate the remaining 1/4 teaspoon of salt. Garnish the ribs with parsley if desired and serve them with the gravy.

Nutrition Facts (per serving)

281	Calories
15g	Fat
13g	Carbs
20g	Protein

Beef Stir-Fry with Baby Bok Choy & Ginger

Prep Time: 25 mins   **Total Time:** 25 mins

Servings: 4   **Yield:** 5 cups

Ingredients

12 ounces beef flank steak, trimmed

1 tablespoon minced fresh ginger

1 ½ teaspoons reduced-sodium soy sauce

1 teaspoon dry sherry plus 1 Tbsp., divided

1 teaspoon cornstarch

1 teaspoon toasted sesame oil

2 tablespoons oyster-flavored sauce, preferably Lee Kum Kee Premium

1 tablespoon vegetable oil

1 pound baby bok choy, trimmed and cut into 2-inch pieces (about 8 cups)

3 tablespoons unsalted chicken broth

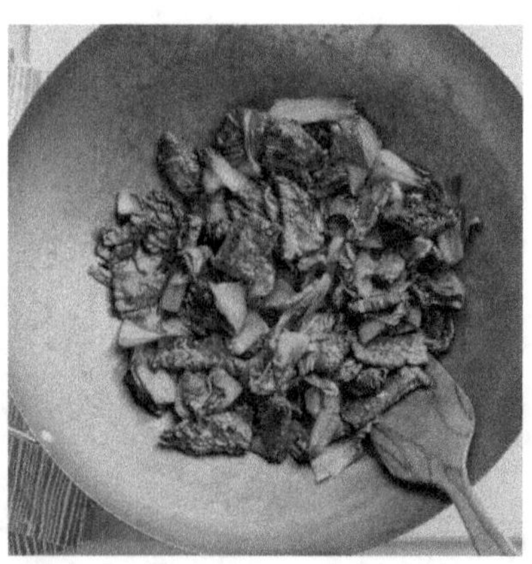

Directions

Cut the beef into 2-inch-wide sections by cutting it across the grain. Cut each strip into 1/4-inch sections by cutting it across the grain. Combine the beef, ginger, soy sauce, 1 tsp sherry and cornstarch are in a medium basin.

Stir until the cornstarch is fully dissolved. Toss the steak in the sesame oil until it is barely coated.

Combine the oyster-flavored sauce and the remaining 1 tablespoon of sherry in a small basin. Set aside.

Place a 14-nch flat-bottomed carbon-steel wok (or a 12-inch stainless-steel skillet) over high heat until a drop of water vaporizes after 1 to 2 seconds of contact. Incorporate vegetable oil by swirling.

Allow the beef to cook undisturbed until it caramelizes, which should take approximately one minute.

Use a metal spatula to stir-fry for 30 seconds to 1 minute or until the food is faintly browned but not fully cooked. Transfer to a platter.

Add the broth and bok choy to the pan. Cover the dish and allow it to cook for 1 to 2 minutes, or until the bok choy greens are a vibrant shade of green and nearly all of the liquid has been absorbed.

Return the meat to the pan, stir in the conserved sauce, and heat for 30 seconds to 1 minute, or until the steak is just cooked through and the bok choy is tender-crisp.

Nutrition Facts (per serving)

247	Calories
13g	Fat
6g	Carbs
26g	Protein

Slow-Cooker Braised Beef with Carrots & Turnips

Prep Time: 40 mins   **Additional Time:** 3 hrs 20 mins   **Total Time:** 4 hrs

Servings: 8   **Yield:** 8 servings

Ingredients

1 tablespoon kosher salt

2 teaspoons ground cinnamon

½ teaspoon ground allspice

½ teaspoon ground pepper

¼ teaspoon ground cloves

3-3 1/2 pounds beef chuck roast, trimmed

2 tablespoons extra virgin olive oil

1 chopped medium onion

3 sliced garlic cloves

1 cup of red wine

1 (28-ounce) can of whole tomatoes, ideally San Marzano

5 medium carrots, sliced into 1 inch chunk

2 medium turnips, peeled and cut into half-inch pieces

Chopped fresh basil for garnish.

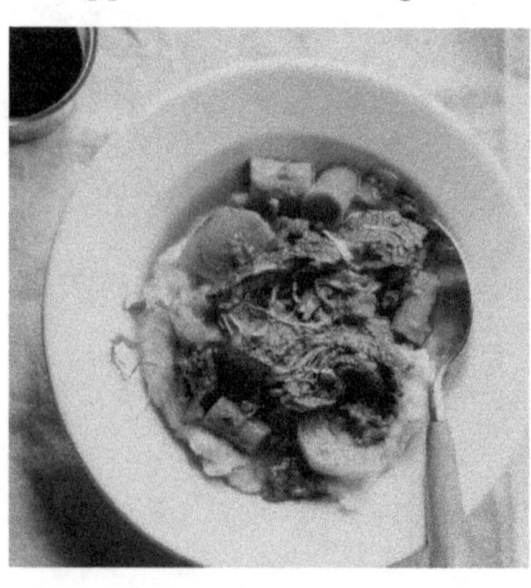

Directions

Salt, cinnamon, allspice, pepper, and cloves should be combined in a small basin. Apply the mixture evenly to the beef.

Heat the oil in a wide skillet over medium heat. Cook the steak for approximately 4 to 5 minutes on each side, or until it is golden brown. Transfer the mixture to a slow cooker that has a capacity of 5 or 6 quarts.

Add the garlic and shallots to the pan. Stir continuously for two minutes. Add the wine and tomatoes (with juice); bring to a boil, breaking up the tomatoes and scraping up any browned fragments.

Add the carrots and turnips to the slow cooker, along with the mélange.

Cover and cook on high for 4 hours or on low for 8 hours.

Remove the steak from the slow cooker and carve it. If desired, garnish the beef with basil and serve it with the sauce and vegetables.

Tips

Active: 40 minutes Slow-cooker time: 4-8 hours

To make ahead: Refrigerate the browned beef (Steps 1-2) and tomato mixture (Step 3) separately for up to 1 day.

Bring the tomato mixture to a boil before adding to the slow cooker.

Nutrition Facts (per serving)

318	Calories
11g	Fat
13g	Carbs
35g	Protein

Rosemary & Garlic-Basted Sirloin Steak

Active Time: 15 mins   **Additional Time:** 35 mins   **Total Time:** 50 mins

Servings: 4   **Yield:** 4 servings

Ingredients

1 pound boneless top sirloin steak, trimmed

1 tablespoon extra-virgin olive oil

¾ teaspoon kosher salt, divided

½ teaspoon ground pepper, divided

4 medium cloves garlic, minced

2 medium shallots, sliced lengthwise

1 ½ tablespoons butter

1 sprig fresh rosemary, plus more for garnish

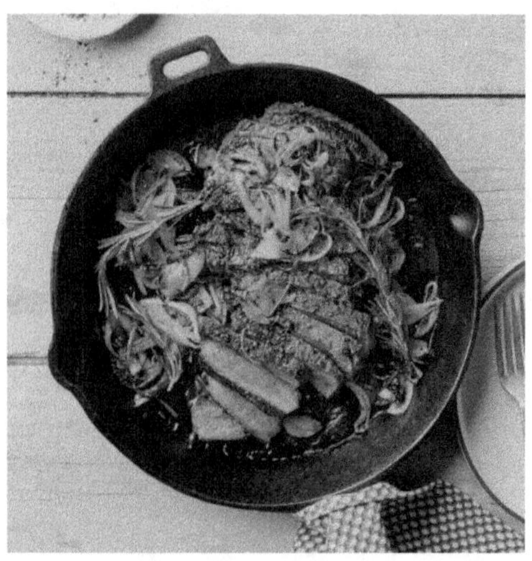

Directions

Allow the meat to remain at room temperature for 30 minutes. Pat the surface dry with paper cloths. Apply oil to the surface, and then season with 1/4 teaspoon pepper and 1/2 teaspoon salt.

Preheat a substantial cast-iron skillet over medium-high fire. Add the meat and allow it to cook for one minute.

Add the garlic, shallots, butter, and rosemary; simmer for 1 minute, tilting the pan gently to collect the butter and drippings on one side.

Apply the butter mixture to the sirloin with a spoon. For medium-rare, cook the steak until an instant-read thermometer registers 125°F, which should take approximately 2 additional minutes.

Baste the steak frequently. Arrange the steak on a clean cutting board and garnish with the shallots, garlic, and rosemary. Cover the dish loosely with foil and allow it to sit for 10 minutes.

The rosemary sprig should be discarded. Place the steak on a serving dish and thinly slice it against the grain.

Drizzle the meat with the drippings from the pan and cutting board. Sprinkle the remaining 1/4 teaspoon of salt and pepper over the dish, and if desired, add more rosemary.

Nutrition Facts (per serving)

216	Calories
12g	Fat
3g	Carbs
23g	Protein

Skillet Steak with Mushroom Sauce

Prep Time: 20 mins   **Additional Time:** 5 mins   **Total Time:** 25 mins

Servings: 4   **Yield:** 4 servings

Ingredients

12 ounces boneless beef top sirloin steak, cut 1 inch thick and trimmed

2 teaspoons salt-free steak grilling seasoning, such as Mrs. Dash®

2 cloves garlic, minced

½ teaspoon salt, divided

2 teaspoons canola oil

6 ounces broccoli, trimmed

2 cups frozen peas

1 teaspoon chopped fresh thyme

3 cups sliced fresh mushrooms

1 cup unsalted beef broth

1 tablespoon whole-grain mustard

2 teaspoons cornstarch

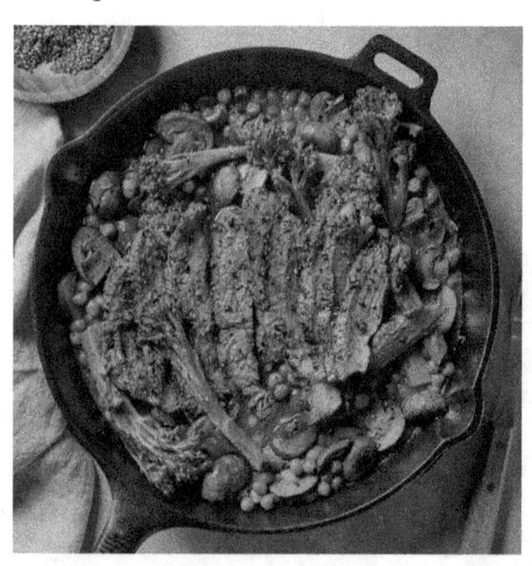

Directions

Preheat the oven to 350° F. Garlic, sirloin seasoning, and 1/4 teaspoon of salt should be sprinkled over the beef. Heat the oil in a 12-inch cast-iron skillet over medium-high heat. Combine the broccoli and the steak.

Cook the broccoli for four minutes, flipping it once (not the sirloin). Arrange peas around the sirloin and sprinkle with thyme. Bake the steak for approximately eight minutes, or until it reaches a medium-rare temperature of 145°F. Transfer the steak and vegetables to a platter, reserving the drippings in the pan. Maintain the temperature by covering it.

Incorporate mushrooms into the drippings of the pan. Stir occasionally while cooking over medium-high heat for three minutes. Combine the broth, mustard, cornstarch, and the remaining ¼ teaspoon of salt in a small bowl or measuring cup.

Pour the mixture into the pan that contains the mushrooms. Stir the mixture until it becomes viscous and bubbly, which should take approximately one to two minutes. Continue to cook while agitating for an additional minute. Serve the sauce alongside the meat and vegetables.

Nutrition Facts (per serving)

231	Calories
7g	Fat
18g	Carbs
26g	Protein

Slow-Cooked Beef with Carrots & Cabbage

Prep Time: 20 mins   **Additional Time:** 4 hrs   **Total Time:** 4 hrs 20 mins

Servings: 2   **Yield:** 2 servings

Ingredients

8 ounces boneless beef chuck pot roast

¼ teaspoon dried oregano, crushed

¼ teaspoon ground cumin

¼ teaspoon paprika

¼ teaspoon ground black pepper

⅛ teaspoon salt

Nonstick cooking spray

3 medium carrots, cut into 2-inch pieces

2 small garlic cloves, minced

⅓ cup lower-sodium beef broth

2 cups coarsely shredded green cabbage

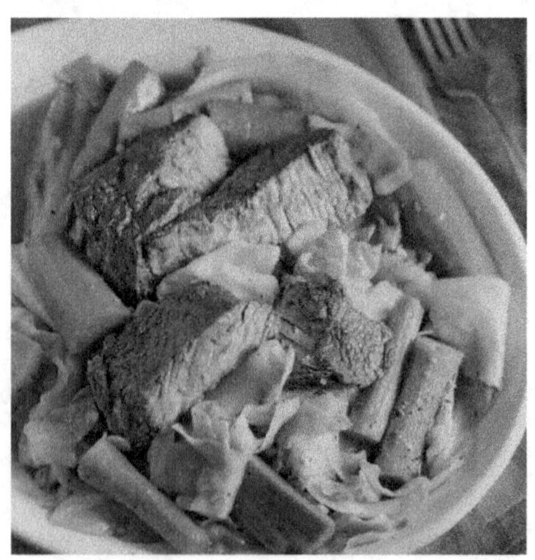

Directions

Trim the fat off the meat. In a small bowl, combine the oregano, cumin, paprika, pepper, and salt.

Sprinkle the mixture evenly over the meat and work the seasoning in with your fingertips. Coat a medium nonstick skillet with cooking spray and heat it over medium heat. Add the meat to the skillet and brown on all sides.

Meanwhile, in a 1 1/2- or 2-quart slow cooker, add the carrots and garlic. Pour broth over the carrots. Top with meat.

Cover and cook for 7 to 8 hours on low heat, or 3 1/2 to 4 hours on high. If no heat setting is available, cook for 5–5 1/2 hours.

At this stage, if you're using the low-heat setting, switch to the high-heat setting. Add cabbage.

Cover and cook for a further 30 minutes. With a slotted spoon, transfer the cabbage, beef, and carrots to a serving plate.

Nutrition Facts (per serving)

214	Calories
5g	Fat
14g	Carbs

28g   Protein

Beef & Bean Sloppy Joes

Prep Time: 20 mins   **Total Time:** 20 mins

Servings: 4   **Yield:** 4 sandwiches

Ingredients

1 tablespoon extra-virgin olive oil

12 ounces 90%-lean ground beef

1 cup no-salt-added black beans, rinsed

1 cup chopped onion

2 teaspoons New Mexico chile powder

½ teaspoon garlic powder

½ teaspoon onion powder

Pinch of cayenne pepper

1 cup no-salt-added tomato sauce

3 tablespoons ketchup

1 tablespoon reduced-sodium   Worcestershire sauce

2 teaspoons spicy brown mustard

1 teaspoon light brown sugar

4 whole-wheat hamburger buns, split and toasted

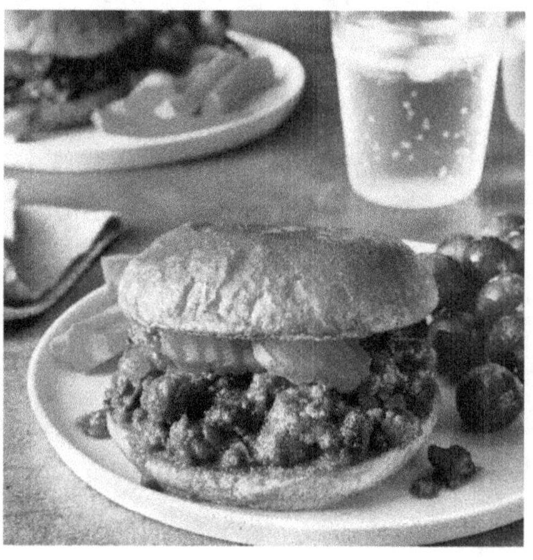

Directions

Heat the oil in a large nonstick skillet over medium-high heat. Heat the meat, breaking it up with a wooden spoon, and add it to the pan. Cook for 3 to 4 minutes, or until it is faintly browned but not fully cooked. Transfer the meat to a medium receptacle using a slotted spoon, reserving the drippings in the pan.

Cook the beans and onion in the pan, stirring frequently, until the onion softens, which should take approximately five minutes.

Stir in the chile powder, garlic powder, onion powder, and cayenne; simmer for approximately 30 seconds, stirring continuously, until the mixture is fragrant. Incorporate the Worcestershire sauce, mustard, brown sugar, ketchup, and tomato sauce.

Return the beef to the pan. The meat should be cooked until it is just cooked through and the sauce has thickened slightly, which should take approximately five minutes. The mixture should be brought to a simmer and stirred frequently. Accompany with pastries.

Nutrition Facts (per serving)

411	Calories
15g	Fat
44g	Carbs
26g	Protein

Slow-Cooker Beef Stroganoff

Prep Time: 30 mins   **Additional Time:** 4 hrs   **Total Time:** 4 hrs 30 mins

Servings: 6   **Yield:** 6 servings

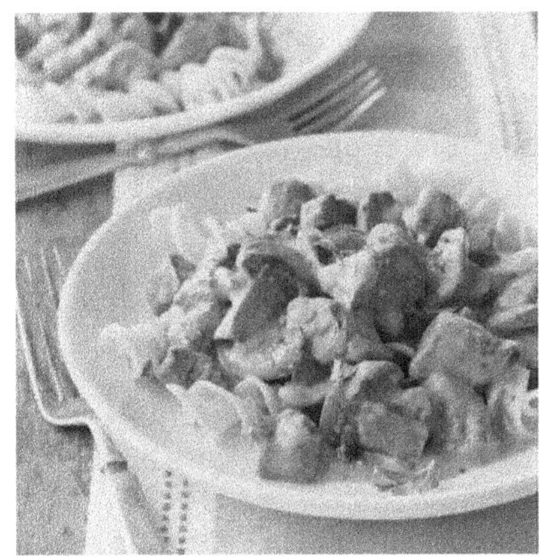

Ingredients

1 ½ pounds of beef stew meat

2 teaspoons of vegetable oil

2 cups of sliced fresh mushrooms

One medium onion, diced (1/2 cup)

2 garlic cloves, minced

½ teaspoon dried oregano, crushed

½ teaspoon salt

¼ teaspoon dried thyme, crushed

¼ teaspoon black pepper

One bay leaf

1 (14.5 ounce) can lower-sodium beef broth

⅓ cup dry sherry or lower-sodium beef broth

1 (8 ounce) carton light sour cream

2 tablespoons cornstarch

2 cups hot cooked noodles

1 snipped fresh parsley

Directions

Trim the fat from beef. Cut the beef into one-inch chunks. In a large skillet, fry meat in heated oil over medium heat, half at a time, until brown. Drain the fat.

In a 3 1/2- or 4-quart slow cooker, combine the mushrooms, onion, garlic, oregano, salt, thyme, pepper, and bay leaf. Include meat. Pour broth and sherry over everything in the crockpot.

Cover and cook on low for 8 to 10 hours or on high for 4 to 5 hours. Remove and discard the bay leaf.

If you're using the low heat setting, switch to the high heat setting. In a medium bowl, combine the sour cream and cornstarch. Gradually incorporate about 1 cup of the heated cooking liquid into the sour cream mixture. Stir the sour cream mixture into the crockpot.

Cover and cook for about 30 minutes more or until thickened. Serve over hot cooked noodles. If desired, sprinkle each serving with parsley.

Tip

For easy cleanup, line your slow cooker with a disposable slow cooker liner. Add ingredients as directed in the recipe. Once your dish is finished cooking, spoon the food out of your slow cooker and simply dispose of the liner. Do not lift or transport the disposable liner with food inside.

Nutrition Facts (per serving)

257	Calories
10g	Fat
14g	Carbs
26g	Protein

Scallion-Ginger Beef & Broccoli

Prep Time: 30 mins   **Total Time:** 30 mins

Servings: 4   **Yield:** 4 servings

Ingredients

⅓ cup reduced-sodium tamari or soy sauce

¼ cup low-sodium chicken broth

2 tablespoons brown sugar

2 tablespoons cornstarch, divided

1 pound sirloin steak, thinly sliced

3 tablespoons peanut or canola oil, divided

6 cups broccoli florets

½ cup sliced scallions, plus more for garnish

1 tablespoon finely grated ginger

1 teaspoon finely grated garlic

2 cups cooked brown rice

Crushed red pepper for garnish

Directions

In a small bowl, whisk together the tamari (or soy sauce), broth, brown sugar, and 1 tablespoon of cornstarch. Toss the meat with the remaining 1 tablespoon cornstarch.

Heat 2 tablespoons oil in a big flat-bottomed wok or cast-iron skillet over medium-high heat.

Cook, stirring once, until the meat is browned, which should take about 4 minutes. Transfer to a clean plate.

Add the broccoli and the remaining 1 tablespoon oil; cook for approximately 2 minutes, turning occasionally, until slightly soft.

Cook, stirring, until the scallions, ginger, and garlic are fragrant, about 30 seconds.

Whisk the tamari mixture and return it to the pan, along with the meat, to heat until the sauce thickens, about 1 minute. Serve over brown rice and garnish with crushed red pepper, if preferred.

Nutrition Facts (per serving)

441	Calories
16g	Fat
43g	Carbs
30g	Protein

Tater Tot Casserole with Beef, Corn & Zucchini

Active Time: 30 mins   **Total Time:** 45 mins

Servings: 6

Ingredients

2 tablespoons extra-virgin olive oil

1 pound lean ground beef

1 small onion, chopped

2 medium zucchini, shredded

1 ½ cups chopped tomatoes, divided

1 cup corn kernels

1 tablespoon chili powder

1 tablespoon Worcestershire sauce

¼ teaspoon salt

1 tablespoon all-purpose flour

1 cup shredded sharp Cheddar cheese, divided

2 cups frozen tater or veggie tots

Cooking spray

Chopped chives for garnish

Directions

Preheat the oven to 450°F.

Heat oil in a large ovenproof skillet over medium-high heat. Combine meat and onion. Cook, breaking up the beef with a wooden spoon, until the onion softens and the beef is no longer pink, about 5 minutes.

Stir in the zucchini, 1 cup tomatoes, corn, chili powder, Worcestershire, and salt; cook for about 3 minutes, or until the zucchini begins to release liquid.

Sprinkle with flour and cook, stirring, until the liquid thickens, about 1 minute more. Remove from heat.

Spread the ingredients in a uniform layer. Sprinkle with 1/2 cup cheese and equally distribute the tots. Spray the tots with cooking spray. Transfer the pan to the oven.

Bake for 15 minutes. Sprinkle the remaining 1/2 cup cheese over the tots and bake for another 5 minutes or until the cheese is melted and golden brown. Garnish with the remaining 1/2 cup tomatoes and chives, if desired.

Nutrition Facts (per serving)

382	Calories
23g	Fat

22g   Carbs   23g   Protein

FISH AND SEAFOOD

1. One-Pot Garlicky Shrimp & Spinach

Active Time: 25 mins   **Total Time:** 25 mins

Servings: 4   **Yield:** 4 cups

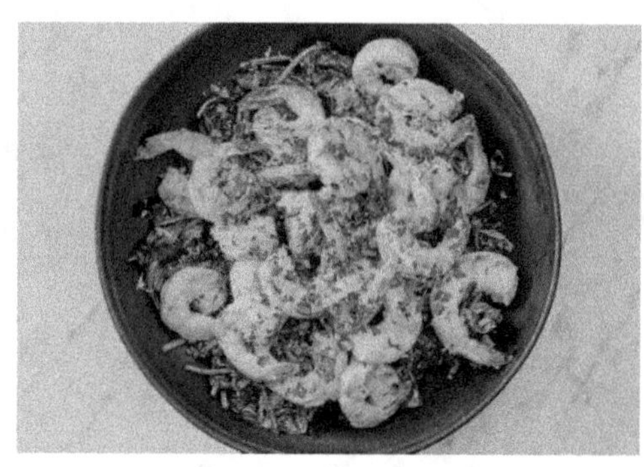

Ingredients

3 tablespoons extra-virgin olive oil, divided

6 medium cloves garlic, sliced, divided

1 pound spinach

¼ teaspoon salt plus 1/8 teaspoon, divided

1 tablespoon lemon juice

1 pound shrimp (21-30 count), peeled and deveined

¼ teaspoon crushed red pepper

1 tablespoon finely chopped fresh parsley

1 ½ teaspoons lemon zest

Directions

1. Heat one tablespoon of oil in a large pot over medium heat. When the garlic starts to brown, add half of it and sauté it for one to two minutes.
2. Add the spinach and 1/4 teaspoon of salt, tossing to coat. Simmer for 3 to 5 minutes,

stirring once or twice, or until mostly wilted. After taking off the heat, stir in the lemon juice. To maintain warmth, transfer to a bowl.

3. After turning up the heat to medium-high, pour the last two teaspoons of oil into the saucepan.

4. Cook for one to two minutes, or until the remaining garlic starts to brown. Incorporate the shrimp, crushed red pepper, and the leftover 1/8 teaspoon of salt.

5. Simmer, stirring occasionally, for an additional 3 to 5 minutes, or until the shrimp are cooked through. Garnish the shrimp with parsley and lemon zest and serve them over spinach.

Nutrition Facts (per serving)

226	Calories
12g	Fat
6g	Carbs
26g	Protein

Walnut-Rosemary Crusted Salmon

Cook Time: 10 mins   **Active Time:** 10 mins   **Total Time:** 20 mins

Servings: 4   **Yield:** 4 serving

Ingredients

2 teaspoons Dijon mustard

1 clove garlic, minced

¼ teaspoon lemon zest

1 teaspoon lemon juice

1 teaspoon chopped fresh rosemary

½ teaspoon honey

½ teaspoon kosher salt

¼ teaspoon crushed red pepper

3 tablespoons panko breadcrumbs

3 tablespoons finely chopped walnuts

1 teaspoon extra-virgin olive oil

1 (1 pound) skinless salmon fillet, fresh or frozen

Olive oil cooking spray

Chopped fresh parsley and lemon wedges for garnish

Directions

Set oven temperature to 425 degrees Fahrenheit. Apply parchment paper to a large baking sheet with a rim.

Mix mustard, garlic, lemon zest, lemon juice, rosemary, honey, salt, and crushed red pepper in a small bowl. Mix the oil, walnuts, and panko together in a separate small bowl.

After the baking sheet is ready, put the fish on it. Cover the fish with the mustard mixture, then top with the panko mixture, pressing to adhere. Apply a thin layer of cooking spray.

Depending on thickness, bake the salmon for 8 to 12 minutes, or until it flakes easily with a fork.

If preferred, serve with lemon wedges and garnish with parsley.

Nutrition Facts (per serving)

222	Calories
12g	Fat
4g	Carbs
24g	Protein

Seasoned Cod

Prep Time: 10 mins   **Cook Time:** 10 mins   **Total Time:** 20 mins

Servings: 8   **Yield:** 8 servings

Ingredients

2 pounds fresh or frozen skinless cod fillets, 3/4- to 1-inch thick

1 teaspoon paprika

½ teaspoon seasoned salt

8 wedges Lemon wedges and/or fresh parsley sprigs

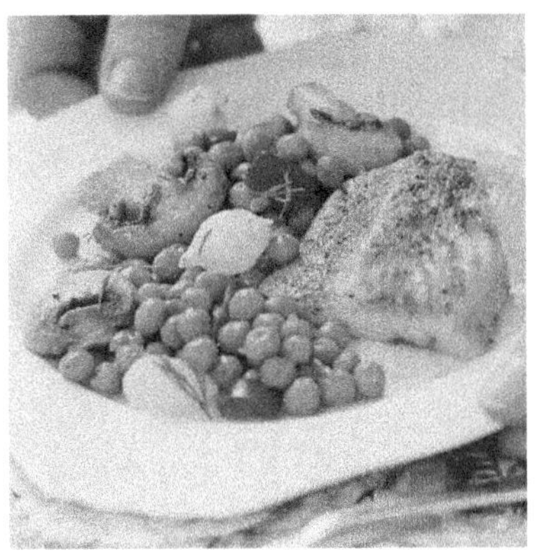

Directions

Preheat the broiler. If you have frozen fish, thaw it. Rinse fish and pat dry with paper towels. In a small bowl, combine the paprika and seasoned salt. Sprinkle the paprika mixture on both sides of the fish fillets. Measure the thickness of the fish.

Place the fish on the broiler pan's oiled, unheated rack. Broil 4 inches from the flame for 4 to 6 minutes per 1/2-inch thickness of salmon, or until readily flaked with a fork. If desired, add lemon wedges and/or parsley sprigs. Makes eight servings.

Microwave Directions: Prepare as specified in Step 1. In a microwave-safe 2-quart square baking dish, put the fish in a single layer. Cover with ventilated plastic wrap. Microwave on 100% power (high) for 5 to 7 minutes, or until the fish readily flakes with a fork, flipping the dish halfway through cooking if required. If desired, add lemon wedges and/or parsley sprigs.

Nutrition Facts (per serving)

| 93 | Calories | 0g | Carbs |
| 1g | Fat | 20g | Protein |

Salmon with Lemon-Herb Orzo & Broccoli

Active Time: 25 mins   **Total Time:** 25 mins

Servings: 4

Ingredients

1 cup orzo (ideally whole-wheat)

2 cups chopped broccoli (about 1/2 head)

3 tablespoons extra virgin olive oil with

1 ¼ pounds skin-on salmon fillet, cut into 4 parts, and pat dry

1/2 teaspoon salt, divided

½ teaspoon ground pepper, divided

4 tablespoons chopped fresh herbs, such as tarragon, chives and/or parsley

2 teaspoons lemon zest

1 tablespoon lemon juice

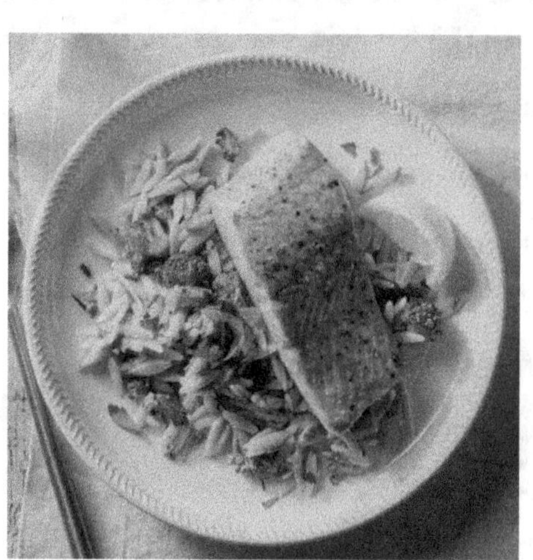

Directions

Bring 2 quarts of water to a boil in a big saucepan. Cook the orzo according to the package guidelines, adding the broccoli for the final minute. Drain and rinse in cool water.

100

Meanwhile, heat 1 1/2 teaspoons of oil in a large nonstick skillet over medium-high heat. Season salmon with 1/4 teaspoon salt and pepper.

Cook, skin side up, until golden brown, 3 to 5 minutes. Flip and cook until the meat is opaque, which should take 3 to 5 minutes depending on thickness.

In a medium bowl, combine 2 tablespoons oil, herbs, lemon zest, lemon juice, and the remaining 1/4 teaspoon each of salt and pepper. Stir in the orzo and broccoli until evenly incorporated.

Serve the orzo mixture with the fish, drizzled with the remaining 1 1/2 tablespoons oil.

Nutrition Facts (per serving)

425	Calories
17g	Fat
32g	Carbs
35g	Protein

Italian Mussels & Pasta

Cook Time: 40 mins   **Total Time:** 40 mins

Servings: 4   **Yield:** 4 servings

Ingredients

8 ounces whole-wheat linguine or spaghetti

¼ cup extra-virgin olive oil

2 large cloves garlic, chopped

1 15-ounce can crushed tomatoes with basil

Big pinch of saffron threads (see Note), soaked in 2 tablespoons water or white wine

2 pounds mussels, cleaned (see Tips)

¾ cup dry white wine

Big pinch of crushed red pepper

¼ teaspoon salt

Freshly ground pepper to taste

¼ cup chopped fresh parsley

1 tablespoon finely grated lemon zest (see Tips)

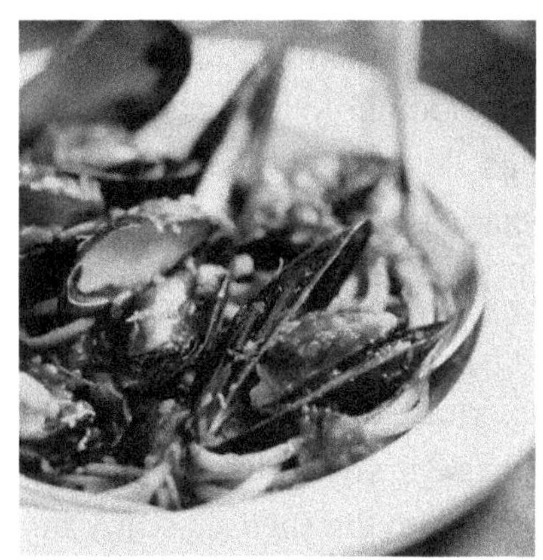

Directions

Heat a big saucepan of water to a boil. Follow the cooking instructions on the pasta package.

After draining, move to a sizable serving bowl. To stay warm, wrap up.

Meanwhile, place a large saucepan over medium heat to warm the oil. Stir and cook for 2 to 3 minutes, or until the garlic is just starting to brown.

Being cautious not to splatter, bring the soaking liquid together with the crushed tomatoes and saffron to a simmer. Simmer, stirring frequently, for about 5 minutes or until slightly thickened.

Meanwhile, place the mussels in a Dutch oven (or large pot) and bring the wine to a boil over high heat.

After you cover and reduce the heat to medium, simmer the mussels for 4 to 6 minutes, or until they open. Transfer the mussels to a large bowl using a slotted spoon. (Toss any mussels that aren't opened.)

Strain the mussel juice into the tomato sauce through a fine-mesh filter. Add the crushed red pepper and simmer over medium heat for one minute.

Add pepper and salt for seasoning. Mix the spaghetti with about half of the sauce. Spoon a little of the remaining sauce over the mussels and divide the spaghetti among four pasta bowls. Garnish with lemon zest and parsley.

Tips

The dried stigma from Crocus sativus, saffron adds flavor and golden color to a variety of Middle Eastern, African and European foods. Soak it in a little water, wine or broth for about 30 minutes before adding to a dish to help release its delicious flavor. Find it in the spice section of supermarkets, gourmet shops or at tienda.com. It will keep in an airtight container for several years.

To clean mussels, rinse very well under cold running water and use a stiff brush to remove any barnacles or grit from the shell. Discard any mussels with broken shells or any whose shells remain open after you tap them lightly. Pull off any fibrous "beard" that might be pinched between the shells; the "beards" of most cultivated mussels are already removed.

A micro plane grater is a great kitchen gadget that seems to be tailor-made for grating citrus zest. It was originally designed to function as a woodworking tool (called a carpenter's rasp). Its razor-sharp edges shave off the zest effortlessly and make it easier to leave the bitter white pith on the fruit. It's the right tool when you want fluffy, very fine citrus zest. Traditional kitchen graters can be used for zesting citrus, too, but they have a tendency to rip and shred the zest, giving a somewhat clumpier, wet result.

Nutrition Facts (per serving)

471	Calories
17g	Fat
56g	Carbs
20g	Protein

Sheet-Pan Chili-Lime Salmon with Potatoes & Peppers

Prep Time: 25 mins   **Total Time:** 25 mins

Servings: 4   **Yield:** 1 serving

Ingredients

1 pound Yukon Gold potatoes, chopped into 3/4-inch chunks

2 tablespoons extra virgin olive oil

¾ teaspoon salt,

¼ teaspoon ground pepper

2 teaspoons of chili powder

1 teaspoon ground cumin

½ teaspoon garlic powder

One lime, zested and quartered

2 medium bell peppers (any color), sliced

1 ¼ pounds center-cut salmon fillet, peeled if preferred, and divided into four parts.

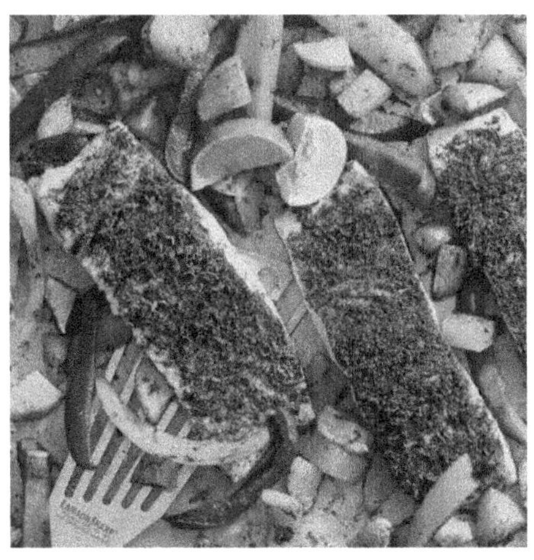

Directions

Set oven temperature to 425 degrees Fahrenheit. Apply cooking spray to a large baking sheet with a rim.

Toss potatoes with 1/4 teaspoon salt, pepper, and 1 tablespoon oil in a medium dish. Place in the prepared pan and bake for fifteen minutes.

Meanwhile, combine the lime zest, chili powder, cumin, garlic powder, and remaining 1/2 teaspoon salt in a another bowl. Toss to coat the bell peppers with the remaining 1 tablespoon oil, 1/2 tablespoon spice combination, and a medium-sized bowl. Apply the remaining spice mixture to the salmon.

Remove the pan from the oven after 15 minutes. Add the peppers and stir until fully mixed. For five minutes, roast. Take out of the oven, reposition some of the veggies, and then put the salmon back in the pan. Bake the fish for 6 to 8 minutes, until it's just done. Accompany with wedges of lime.

Nutrition Facts (per serving)

405	Calories
17g	Fat
26g	Carbs

35g	Protein

Spicy Jerk Shrimp

Active Time: 35 mins   **Total Time:** 50 mins

Servings: 4   **Yield:** 4 servings

Ingredients

1 ½ pounds fresh or frozen large shrimp in shells

4 (1/4 inch thick) slices peeled and cored fresh pineapple, halved

2 cups bite-size strips red sweet pepper

2 cups sliced red onions

1 fresh jalapeño chile pepper, halved lengthwise, seeded and sliced (see Tip)

2 tablespoons olive oil

1 tablespoon Jamaican jerk seasoning

½ cup coarsely snipped fresh cilantro

1 ⅓ cups hot cooked brown rice

Lime wedges

Directions

Thaw any frozen shrimp you may have. Set oven temperature to 425 degrees Fahrenheit. Two 15-by-10-inch baking pans should be lined with foil.

Peel and devein shrimp, if preferred, leaving the tails in place. After rinsing, pat shrimp dry.

In an extra-large bowl, toss shrimp with the next six ingredients (through jerk seasoning) until completely covered. Distribute the blend among the ready pans. Roast the shrimp for fifteen minutes, or until they become opaque.

Garnish with cilantro and serve with lime wedges and brown rice.

Tips

Oils from chile peppers can irritate the skin and eyes. Put on rubber or plastic gloves before handling them.

Nutrition Facts (per serving)

351	Calories
9g	Fat
37g	Carbs

34g   Protein

Provencal Baked Fish with Roasted Potatoes & Mushrooms

Prep Time: 15 mins   **Additional Time:** 45 mins   **Total Time:** 1 hr

Servings: 4   **Yield:** 4 servings

Ingredients

1 pound Yukon Gold or red potatoes, cubed

1 pound mushrooms (shiitake, cremini, oyster or other fresh mushrooms), trimmed and sliced

2 tablespoons extra-virgin olive oil, divided

¼ teaspoon salt

¼ teaspoon ground pepper

2 cloves garlic, peeled and sliced

14 ounces halibut, grouper or cod fillet, cut into 4 portions

4 tablespoons lemon juice

1 teaspoon herbes de Provence

Fresh thyme for garnish

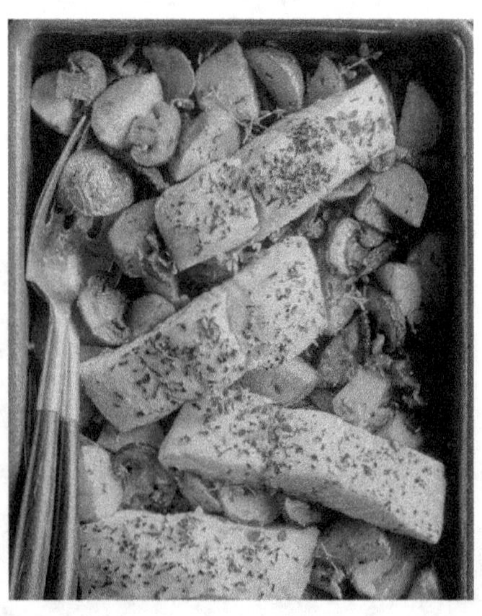

Directions

Set oven temperature to 425 degrees Fahrenheit.

Add the potatoes, mushrooms, 1 tablespoon oil, salt, and pepper to a large mixing bowl. Turn out onto a 9 x 13-inch baking sheet. Bake the veggies for thirty to forty minutes, or until they are somewhat soft.

Add the garlic after stirring the veggies. Put the fish on top. Pour in the remaining 1 tablespoon oil and lemon juice. Add a little Herbes de Provence. Bake the salmon for ten to fifteen minutes, or until it is flake-able and opaque throughout. If desired, garnish with thyme.

Nutrition Facts (per serving)

276	Calories
9g	Fat
25g	Carbs
24g	Protein

Skillet Gnocchi with Shrimp & Asparagus

Cook Time: 30 mins   **Total Time:** 30 mins

Servings: 4   **Yield:** 4 servings, about 1 1/2 cups each

Ingredients

1 tablespoon plus 2 teaspoons extra-virgin olive oil, divided

1 16-ounce package shelf-stable gnocchi

½ cup sliced shallots

1 bunch asparagus (about 1 pound), trimmed and cut into thirds

¾ cup reduced-sodium chicken broth

1 pound raw shrimp (26-30 per pound), peeled and deveined, tails left on if desired

¼ teaspoon freshly ground pepper

Pinch of salt

2 tablespoons lemon juice

⅓ cup grated Parmesan cheese

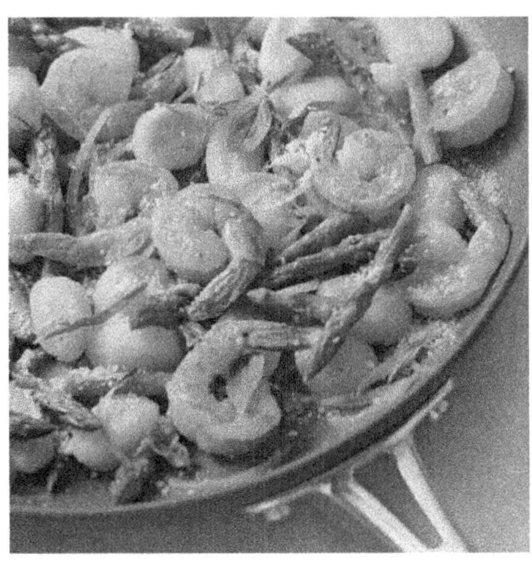

Directions

Heat 1 tablespoon oil in a large nonstick skillet over medium heat. Cook the gnocchi, tossing frequently, until plumped and brown in places, about 6 to 10 minutes. Transfer to a bowl.

Cook the remaining 2 tablespoons oil and shallots in the pan over medium heat, stirring, until they begin to brown, about 1 to 2 minutes. Stir in the asparagus and broth. Cover and heat for 3-4 minutes, or until the asparagus is barely tender. Add the shrimp, pepper, and salt; cover and boil for 3 to 4 minutes, or until the shrimp is pink and just cooked through.

Return the gnocchi to the skillet and add the lemon juice, stirring until cooked through, about 2 minutes. Remove from heat, sprinkle with cheese, cover, and set aside for about 2 minutes to allow the cheese to melt.

Nutrition Facts (per serving)

466	Calories
9g	Fat
65g	Carbs
32g	Protein

Herby Fish with Wilted Greens & Mushrooms

Prep Time: 25 mins　　　　**Total Time:** 25 mins

Servings: 4　　　　**Yield:** 4 servings

Ingredients

3 tablespoons olive oil, divided

½ large sweet onion, sliced

3 cups sliced cremini mushrooms

2 cloves garlic, sliced

4 cups chopped kale

1 medium tomato, diced

2 teaspoons Mediterranean Herb Mix, divided

1 tablespoon lemon juice

½ teaspoon salt, divided

½ teaspoon ground pepper, divided

4 (4 ounce) cod, sole, or tilapia fillets

Chopped fresh parsley, for garnish

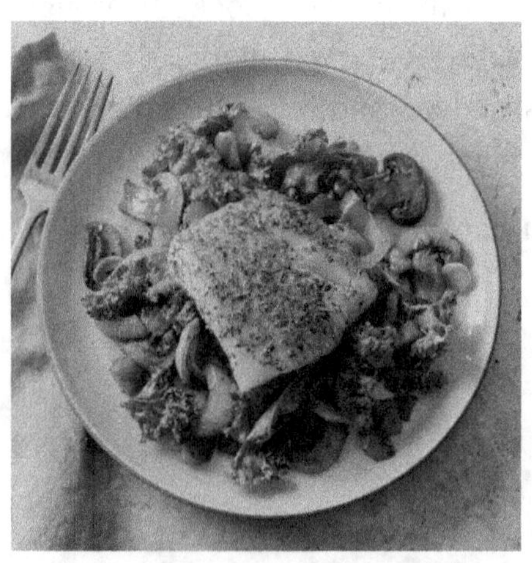

Directions

Heat 1 tablespoon of oil in a large saucepan over medium heat. Cook the onion until it is transparent, stirring occasionally, which should take approximately 3 to 4 minutes.

Cook the mushrooms until they release moisture and begin to brown, stirring intermittently, for approximately 4 to 6 minutes. Combine kale, tomato, and one teaspoon of the herb mixture. Cook for approximately 5 to 7 minutes, stirring intermittently, until the mushrooms are tender and the kale has wilted.

Mix in lemon juice and 1/4 teaspoon of each salt and pepper. Withdraw from the heat source, conceal, and maintain a comfortable temperature.

Sprinkle the fish with the remaining 1/4 teaspoon of salt and pepper and 1 teaspoon of the herb mixture.

Heat the remaining 2 tablespoons of oil in a large nonstick skillet over medium-high heat. The fish should be cooked until the flesh is opaque, which typically takes 2 to 4 minutes per side, depending on its thickness.

Transfer the fish to a serving platter or four dishes. Place the vegetables on top and around the salmon; if desired, add parsley as a garnish.

108

Nutrition Facts (per serving)

214	Calories
11g	Fat
11g	Carbs
18g	Protein

Oven-Fried Fish & Chips

Cook Time: 25 mins   **Additional Time:** 20 mins   **Total Time:** 45 mins

Servings: 4   **Yield:** 16 to 2 oz. fish & cups chips

Ingredients

Use canola or olive oil cooking spray

1 1/2 pounds of russet potatoes, cleaned and sliced into 1/4-inch-thick wedges

4 tsp canola oil

1 1/2 tablespoons Cajun or Creole seasoning, divided

2 cups cornflakes

¼ cup all-purpose flour,

¼ teaspoon salt

2 large egg whites

1 pound of cod or haddock chopped into 4 parts.

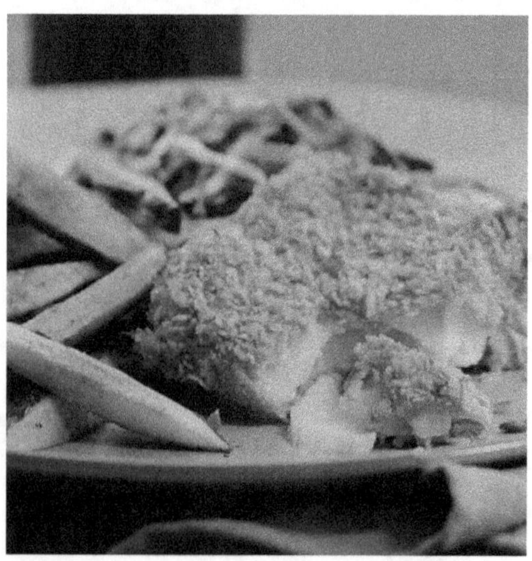

Directions

Preheat the oven to 425 degrees F, with racks in the upper and lower thirds. Spray a large baking sheet with cooking spray. Place a wire rack on another large baking sheet and cover with cooking spray.

Place the potatoes in a colander. Rinse thoroughly with cold water and dry entirely with paper towels.

Combine the potatoes, oil, and 3/4 teaspoon Cajun (or Creole) seasoning in a large mixing basin. Spread on the baking sheet without a rack. Bake for 30 to 35 minutes on the lower oven rack, rotating once every 10 minutes, until soft and brown.

Meanwhile, finely ground the cornflakes in a food processor or blender, or crush them in a sealable plastic bag. Transfer to a shallow dish.

In another shallow dish, combine the flour, remaining 3/4 teaspoon Cajun (or Creole) seasoning, and salt; in a third shallow dish, combine the egg whites.

Dredge the fish in the flour mixture, then dip it in egg white and coat it all over with ground cornflakes. Place on the prepared wire rack. Spray both sides of the breaded fish with cooking spray.

Bake the fish on the upper oven rack for about 20 minutes, or until opaque in the center and the breading is golden brown and crispy.

Tips

Overfishing and trawling have drastically reduced the number of cod in the U.S. and Canadian Atlantic Ocean and destroyed its sea floor. For sustainably fished cod, choose U.S. Pacific cod or Atlantic cod from Iceland and the northeast Arctic. For more information, visit Monterey Bay Aquarium Seafood Watch at seafoodwatch.org.

Easy cleanup: Recipes that require cooking spray can leave behind a sticky residue that can be hard to clean. To save time and keep your baking sheet looking fresh, line it with a layer of foil before you apply the cooking spray.

Nutrition Facts (per serving)

323	Calories
5g	Fat
46g	Carbs
23g	Protein

Shrimp-Stuffed Pasta Shells

Prep Time: 45 mins   **Additional Time:** 40 mins   **Total Time:** 1 hr 25 mins

Servings: 6   **Yield:** 6 servings

Ingredients

1 pound fresh or frozen large shrimp in shells

12 dried jumbo shell macaroni

1 medium red sweet pepper, chopped

½ cup chopped sweet onion

1 tablespoon olive oil

3 cloves garlic, minced

⅓ cup dry white wine or reduced-sodium chicken broth

¾ cup reduced-sodium chicken broth

¼ cup flour

2 cups fat-free milk

8 ounces cooked crabmeat, coarsely chopped, or good-quality canned lump crabmeat, drained

2 tablespoons snipped fresh basil

1 tablespoon snipped fresh chives

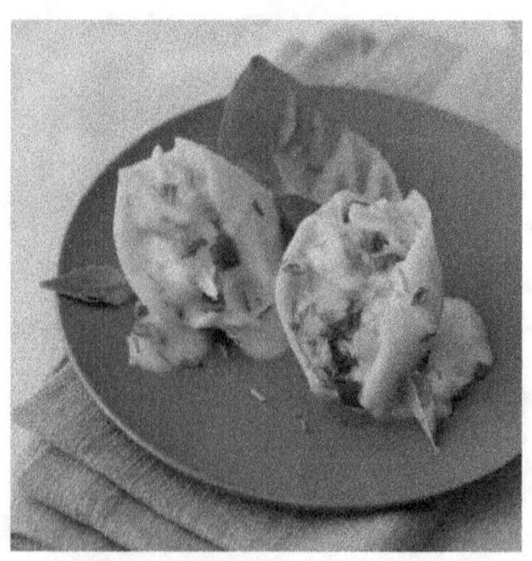

Directions

Thaw any frozen shrimp you may have. Shrimp should be peeled and deveined, then rinsed in cold water and dried with paper towels. Roughly chop the shrimp and reserve. In the meantime, prepare the pasta as directed on the package and then drain. Drain once more after rinsing with cold water.

Set oven temperature to 350 degrees. The sweet pepper and onion should be sautéed in hot oil in a large nonstick skillet over medium heat for five minutes, rotating occasionally.

Put shrimp in. Stirring occasionally, cook for a further two to three minutes, or until the shrimp are opaque. Pour the combination of shrimp into a bowl. Garlic is added to the same skillet to create the sauce. Stir and cook for 30 seconds. Take the skillet off of the burner.

After a minute or two, or when most of the wine has evaporated, return the skillet to the heat and continue cooking, scraping up any browned bits from the bottom. Mix the flour and 3/4 cup of broth together in a small bowl. Pour the milk into the skillet and immediately add all of the ingredients. Cook, stirring, until bubbly and thickened.

Add the crab and 2/3 cup of the sauce to the shrimp mixture and stir. After uniformly filling the baked shells with the shrimp mixture, transfer them to a 2-quart square baking dish. Cover the shells with the remaining sauce.

Bake, covered, for thirty to thirty-five minutes, or until cooked through. Give it a ten-minute rest. Before serving, toss in the chives and basil. Present in shallow serving trays.

Nutrition Facts (per serving)

317	Calories
5g	Fat
33g	Carbs
31g	Protein

Peppery Barbecue-Glazed Shrimp with Vegetables & Orzo

Prep Time: 30 mins   **Total Time:** 30 mins

Servings: 4   **Yield:** 8 cups

Ingredients

1 pound peeled and deveined jumbo shrimp, thawed if frozen (see Tip)

1 teaspoon paprika

½ teaspoon garlic powder

½ teaspoon dried oregano, crushed

¼ teaspoon ground pepper

⅛ teaspoon cayenne pepper

1 cup whole-grain orzo

3 scallions

2 tablespoons olive oil, divided

2 cups coarsely chopped zucchini

1 cup coarsely chopped bell pepper

½ cup thinly sliced celery

1 cup cherry tomatoes, halved

½ teaspoon salt

2 tablespoons barbecue sauce

Lemon wedges for serving

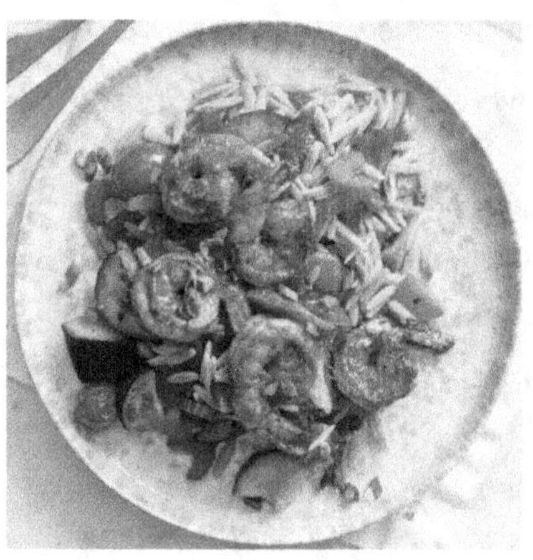

Directions

Transfer the shrimp to a medium-sized bowl. Combine the paprika, cayenne, oregano, garlic powder, and pepper in a small bowl. After tossing the shrimp to coat, sprinkle the spice mixture over them and put them aside.

Bring a large pot of water to a boil. Cook the orzo as directed on the package, then drain. Take back the heated pot, cover, and maintain the warmth.

Meanwhile, cut the green and white parts off of the scallions. In a medium skillet set over medium-high heat, heat 1 tablespoon of oil.

Add the bell pepper, celery, zucchini, and scallion whites and cook, stirring occasionally, until the vegetables are crisp-tender, about 5 minutes.

Simmer for a further two to three minutes, or until the tomatoes are tender. Add the orzo to the pot with the vegetables. Stir in salt to combine.

114

Heat the remaining tablespoon of oil in the same skillet over medium heat. Cook for 4 to 6 minutes, rotating once, or until the shrimp are opaque. Pour on some BBQ sauce. Cook, stirring, for 1 minute, or until all of the shrimp is coated.

Present the shrimp alongside the vegetable mixture. If desired, serve with lemon wedges and garnish with scallion leaves.

Tips

Frozen shrimp thaws quickly. Place frozen shrimp in a large bowl with ice water. Let settle for 20 minutes.

Nutrition Facts (per serving)

360	Calories
9g	Fat
41g	Carbs
30g	Protein

Provencal Fish Fillets

Prep Time: 20 mins   **Additional Time:** 5 mins   **Total Time:** 25 mins

Servings: 4   **Yield:** 4 fillets

Ingredients

4 (4 ounce) fresh or frozen skinless cod, catfish, Pollock, or tilapia fish fillets, 1/2 to 1 inch thick

1 tablespoon olive oil

1 medium onion, thinly sliced

2 cloves garlic, minced

1 (14.5 ounce) can whole tomatoes, drained and chopped

2 teaspoons chopped fresh thyme or 1/2 teaspoon dried, crushed

8 oil-cured Greek olives, pitted and halved, or 8 pitted ripe olives, halved

1 teaspoon capers, drained

4 sprigs Fresh thyme sprigs

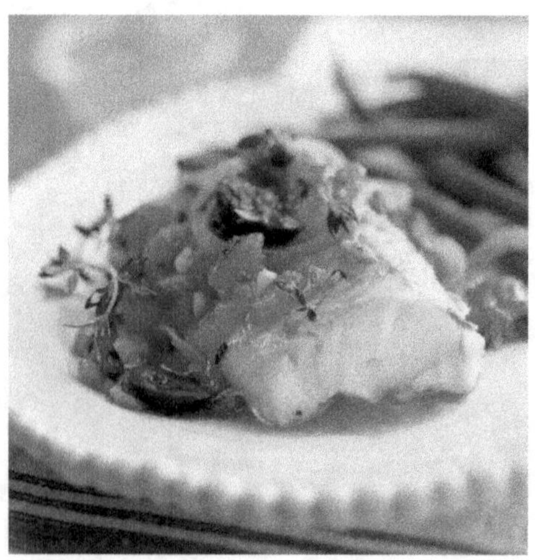

Directions

Thaw frozen seafood. Rinse the fish and pat it dry with paper napkins. Set aside.

Heat oil in a small saucepan over medium heat. When the onion and garlic are added, allow them to simmer for approximately five minutes or until they are tender, stirring occasionally. Combine capers, olives, thyme, and tomatoes. Heat the mixture until it reaches boiling point, and then reduce the heat to medium. Allow the mixture to simmer in the open for approximately 10 minutes, or until the majority of the liquid has dissipated.

In the interim, preheat the broiler. Determine the girth of the fish. Place the fish on a greased, unheated tray in a broiler pan that has been coated with foil, ensuring that any thin edges are tucked under.

Broil the fish at a height of 3 to 4 inches from the flame for 4 to 6 minutes per 1/2-inch thickness, or until it is easily divided with a fork. If the fillets are 1 inch thick, rotate them once. Serve with the sauce and, if desired, garnish with fresh thyme fronds.

Nutrition Facts (per serving)

161	Calories
5g	Fat
7g	Carbs
21g	Protein

116

Alaskan Cod Chowder

Cook Time: 45 mins   **Total Time:** 45 mins

Servings: 6   **Yield:** 6 servings

Ingredients

3 tablespoons extra-virgin olive oil

1 cup diced onion

1 cup diced celery

½ cup all-purpose flour

1 tablespoon Worcestershire sauce

¾ teaspoon reduced-sodium Old Bay seasoning

¼ teaspoon salt

¼ teaspoon ground pepper

4 cups reduced-sodium fish or seafood stock

1 cup whole milk

3 cups diced red potatoes

2 cups chopped green beans

1 pound Alaskan cod (see Tip), cut into 1-inch pieces

Chopped fresh dill for garnish

Chopped plum tomatoes for garnish

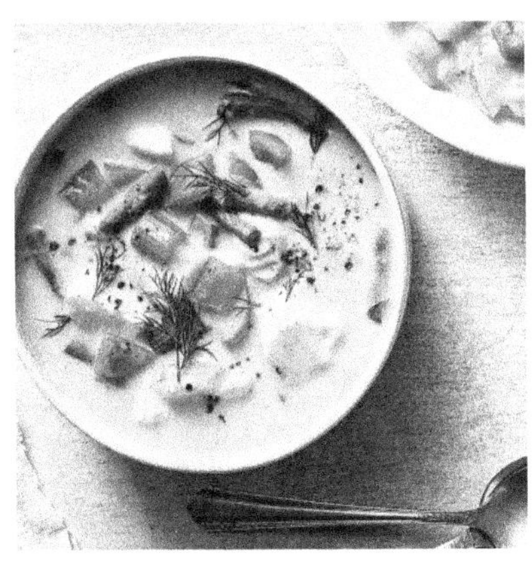

Directions

Heat the oil in a big pot over medium heat. Cook, stirring regularly, until the onion and celery soften and begin to brown, about 3 to 6 minutes.

Sprinkle the flour, Worcestershire sauce, Old Bay seasoning, salt, and pepper over the vegetables and simmer for another minute, stirring.

Add the fish (or seafood) stock and milk; bring to a slow boil while stirring constantly.

Stir in the potatoes and green beans; come to a boil. Simmer, stirring occasionally, until the potatoes are soft, about 12 to 15 minutes.

Cook, tossing regularly, until the cod is cooked through, about 2 to 4 minutes. Serve with dill and tomatoes, if desired.

Tips

Our favorite sustainable cod is U.S. Pacific cod from Alaskan waters; Atlantic cod (sometimes called scrod) from Iceland and the northeast Arctic are also sustainable choices. For more information about choosing sustainable seafood, visit seafoodwatch.org.

To make ahead: Cover and refrigerate for up to 3 days, slowly reheat over medium-low or microwave on Medium power.

Nutrition Facts (per serving)

270	Calories
9g	Fat
29g	Carbs
19g	Protein

Vegan and Vegetarian

1. Chickpea Pasta with Mushrooms & Kale

Active Time: 30 mins   **Total Time:** 30 mins

Servings: 4

Ingredients

8 ounces chickpea rotini *or* penne (see Tip)

¼ cup extra-virgin olive oil

2 large cloves garlic, sliced

Pinch of crushed red pepper

8 cups chopped kale

8 ounces cremini mushrooms, quartered

½ teaspoon dried thyme

½ teaspoon salt

Grated Parmesan cheese for serving (optional)

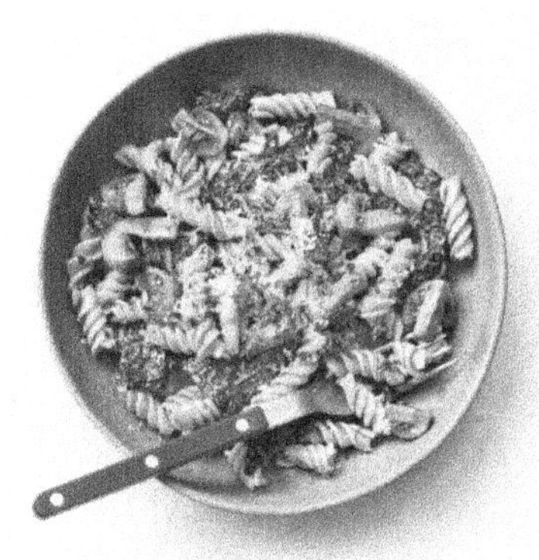

Directions

Follow the cooking instructions on the pasta package. After draining, set one cup of the cooking water aside.

Meanwhile, place a large skillet over medium heat with the oil. Simmer for about a minute, stirring once, or until the crushed red pepper and garlic are fragrant.

Simmer for approximately five minutes, stirring periodically, or until the vegetables are soft.

Add enough of the set-aside water to coat the pasta, then swirl and boil for an additional minute to ensure it's well combined and cooked.

Before serving, top with Parmesan cheese, if desired.

Tip:

I chose chickpea pasta for this dish instead of whole-wheat because it's packed with tons of fiber, protein and nutrients—some brands provide more than 40% of your daily recommended fiber, plus 20 grams of protein per serving. Look for it with other gluten-free pastas.

Nutrition Facts (per serving)

340	Calories
18g	Fat
38g	Carbs
17g	Protein

Butternut Squash & Black Bean Enchiladas

Active Time: 25 mins   **Total Time:** 45 mins

Servings: 4

Ingredients

3 tablespoons extra-virgin olive oil, divided

3 cups diced peeled butternut squash

2 medium poblano peppers, seeded and chopped

1 medium onion, chopped

1 (14 ounce) can no-salt-added black beans, rinsed

4 tablespoons chopped fresh cilantro, divided, plus more for serving

1 tablespoon ancho chile powder

8 corn tortillas, warmed

1 (10-ounce) can enchilada sauce (see Tip)

½ cup shredded Monterey Jack cheese

2 cups shredded cabbage

1 tablespoon lime juice

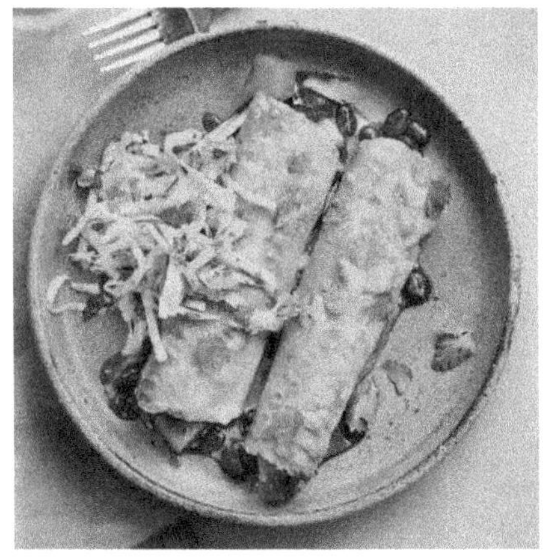

Directions

Preheat the oven to 425°F. Spread cooking spray on a 7 by 11-inch baking dish.

In a big skillet over medium heat, heat two tablespoons of oil. Cook the squash, covered, tossing regularly, for 8 to 10 minutes, or until it's tender and lightly browned.

Cook, uncovered, for about 5 minutes, or until the peppers and onion are tender. Every now and then, stir.

Take off the heat source and combine the beans with two teaspoons of cilantro and chili powder. Give it five minutes to cool.

Roll each tortilla after stuffing it with about 1/2 cup of the squash mixture. Fold seam side down and place in the prepared baking dish. Spoon enchilada sauce over top.

Cover with foil and sprinkle with cheese. Bake, uncovered, until bubbling, about 15 minutes. Take off the foil and bake for a further five minutes.

In the meantime, mix the cabbage, 2 tablespoons of cilantro, lime juice, and the remaining tablespoon of oil.

Garnish the enchiladas with extra cilantro if desired and serve them with the slaw.

Tip:

Store-bought enchilada sauce is a fast and easy way to add a ton of flavor to a dish, but it can be high in sodium, so look for one that has less than 300 milligrams per serving.

Nutrition Facts (per serving)

428	Calories
17g	Fat
58g	Carbs
13g	Protein

Red Lentil Soup with Saffron

Active Time: 20 mins   **Total Time:** 40 mins

Servings: 8

Ingredients

3 tablespoons extra-virgin olive oil

2 medium carrots, finely diced

2 stalks celery, finely diced

1 large onion, finely diced

3 cloves garlic, minced

1 tablespoon tomato paste

½ teaspoon ground cumin

¼ teaspoon crushed saffron threads

¼ teaspoon ground turmeric

4 cups low-sodium no-chicken *or* chicken broth

1 ½ cups water, plus more as needed

1 pound red lentils (2 cups), picked over and rinsed

5 ounces spinach, coarsely chopped

1 teaspoon kosher salt

1 teaspoon ground pepper

Plain yogurt & chopped fresh mint for garnish

Directions

In a big, heavy saucepan, warm the oil over medium heat. Simmer for 7 to 10 minutes, or until the carrots, celery, and onion start to get tender. (Avoid browning.)

Add the turmeric, saffron, cumin, garlic, and tomato paste. Simmer for one minute.

Add the lentil, spinach, water, broth, salt, and pepper. Heat through to a simmer.

Reduce the heat to a simmer, cover, and cook for 15 to 20 minutes, stirring now and then to avoid sticking, or until the lentils and vegetables are tender. If extra water is needed, add it.

Garnish with yogurt and mint if preferred.

Nutrition Facts (per serving)

280	Calories
7g	Fat
42g	Carbs
15g	Protein

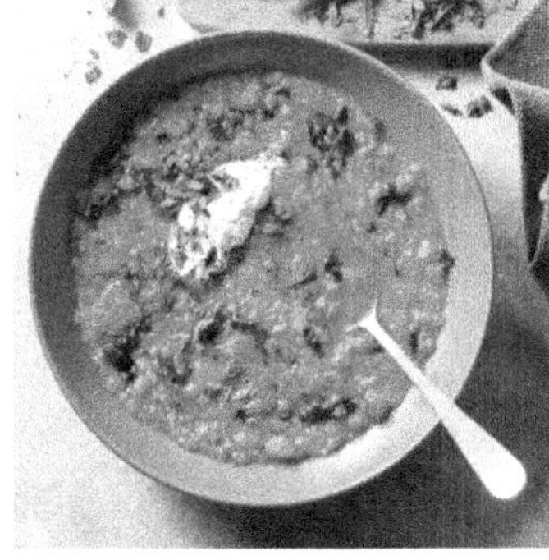

Cauliflower Fajita Skillet

Active Time: 15 mins   **Total Time:** 45 mins

Servings: 6

Ingredients

1 medium head cauliflower, trimmed and thinly sliced

1 medium red bell pepper, sliced

1 medium onion, sliced

3 tablespoons extra-virgin olive oil

1 ½ teaspoons chili powder

1 teaspoon ground cumin

½ teaspoon ground coriander

½ teaspoon salt

¼ teaspoon ground pepper

½ cup pico de gallo

¼ cup chopped pickled jalapeño peppers

Chopped fresh cilantro for garnish

1 14-ounce can light-in-sodium refried beans, warmed

12 corn tortillas, warmed

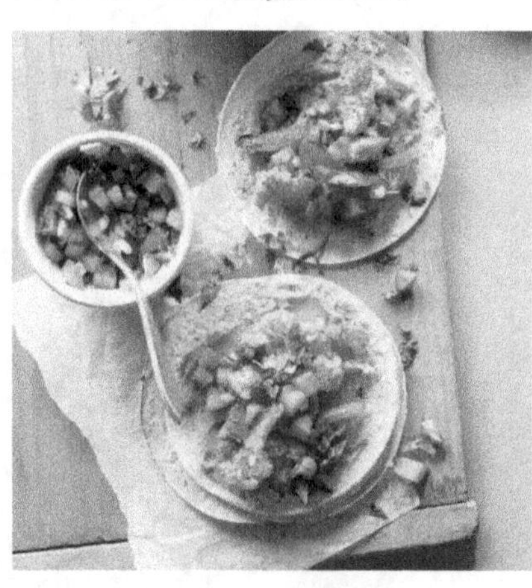

Directions

Place a rack in the top third of the oven and a large cast-iron skillet on it. Preheat to 425°F.

Toss cauliflower, bell pepper, onion, and oil in a medium bowl until coated. Toss with chili powder, cumin, coriander, salt, and pepper until evenly coated. Carefully place the mixture in the hot pan.

Roast, tossing once, until the vegetables are soft, about 30 minutes.

Set the broiler to high. Broil the vegetables for approximately 2 minutes, or until gently browned.

Optional garnishes include pico de gallo, jalapeños, and cilantro. Serve alongside refried beans and tortillas.

Nutrition Facts (per serving)

302	Calories
11g	Fat
48g	Carbs
9g	Protein

Sheet-Pan Balsamic-Parmesan Roasted Chickpeas & Vegetables

Prep Time: 15 mins   **Additional Time:** 25 mins   **Total Time:** 40 mins

Servings: 4   **Yield:** 4 cups

Ingredients

1 (15 ounce) can no-salt-added chickpeas, rinsed

8 ounces multicolored baby carrots with tops, trimmed and peeled

2 bunches spring onions, tops removed and bulbs halved lengthwise

6 tablespoons extra-virgin olive oil, divided

¼ teaspoon salt, divided

8 ounces asparagus, cut into 2-inch pieces

½ cup grated Parmesan cheese

2 tablespoons balsamic vinegar

1 teaspoon honey

½ teaspoon Dijon mustard

½ teaspoon ground pepper

1 teaspoon fresh thyme leaves

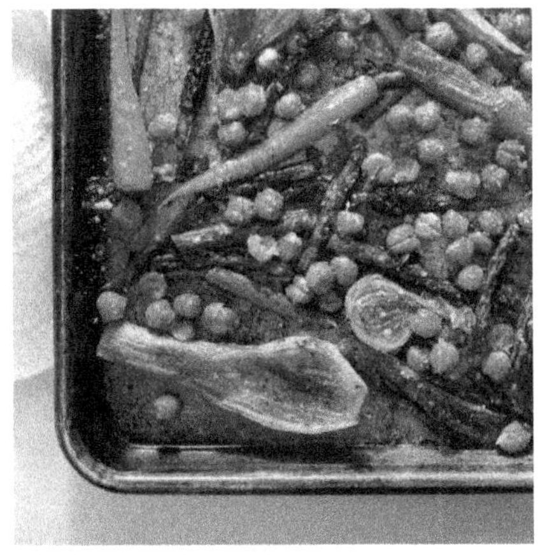

Directions

Raise the oven to 400 degrees F and put a big baking sheet with a lip on the middle rack. Place more paper towels on top of another baking sheet.

Spread the chickpeas out on the paper towels. Use more paper towels to rub off the skins, then throw away the skins.

Get a big bowl and put the chickpeas in it. Throw in the spring onions, carrots, 3 tablespoons of oil, and 1/8 teaspoon of salt. Mix everything together.

Put it on the hot baking sheet in a single layer. For about 30 minutes, toss the veggies every few minutes and add the asparagus for the last 10 minutes of cooking. Roast until the vegetables are golden brown and soft.

Spread the Parmesan cheese out evenly over the vegetables, and roast for another 5 minutes, or until the cheese melts.

In a small bowl, mix the vinegar, honey, mustard, pepper, the last 3 tablespoons of oil, and 1/8 teaspoon of salt. Pour the balsamic sauce over the vegetables, and then top them with thyme leaves. Serve right away.

Nutrition Facts (per serving)

399	Calories
24g	Fat

34g   Carbs   12g   Protein

Sweet Potato-Black Bean Burgers

Prep Time: 15 mins   **Additional Time:** 30 mins   **Total Time:** 45 mins

Servings: 4   **Yield:** 4 burgers

Ingredients

2 cups of sweet potato gratin

Half a cup of old-fashioned rolled oats

1 cup black beans, cleaned and without salt

1/2 cup of chopped scallions

1/4 cup of vegan mayonnaise

1 tablespoon tomato paste with no salt added

1 big pinch of curry powder

1/8 teaspoon of salt

1/2 cup plain almond milk yogurt that hasn't been sweetened

2 tablespoons of fresh dill, cut up

2 tablespoons of juice from lemon

2 tablespoons of olive oil that isn't refined

4 hamburger buns made from whole wheat, toasted1 slice of cucumber, cut very thinly

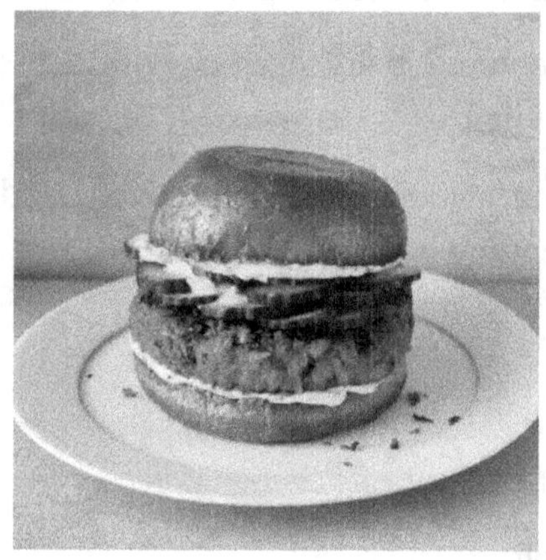

Directions

Use paper towels to squeeze the chopped sweet potato to get rid of extra water, then put it in a big bowl.

Pulse the oats in a food processor until they are very small. Then, add them to the bowl with the sweet potatoes.

In a bowl, mix together the beans, onions, mayonnaise, tomato paste, curry powder, and salt. Use your hands to mash the ingredients together.

Make four patties that are 1/2 inch thick. Put the patties on a plate and put them in the fridge for 30 minutes.

Put yogurt, dill, and lemon juice in a small bowl and mix them together. Set the bowl away.

Warm up the oil in a big cast-iron pan over medium-high heat. Put in the patties and cook for about 3 minutes on each side until they turn golden brown.

Put the same amount of yogurt sauce on both halves of the bun.

Place a burger and cucumber slices on top of each bottom bun half, then put the top bun halves back on.

Tips

To make ahead: Prepare patties (Step 1); wrap and refrigerate for up to 2 days.

Nutrition Facts (per serving)

454	Calories
22g	Fat
54g	Carbs
12g	Protein

Chipotle-Lime Cauliflower Taco Bowls

Prep Time: 20 mins   **Additional Time:** 20 mins   **Total Time:** 40 mins

Servings: 4   **Yield:** 4 bowls

Ingredients

¼ cup lime juice (from about two limes)

1 to 2 cup chopped chipotles in adobo sauce (see Tip)

Two cloves of garlic and one tablespoon of honey

½ teaspoon of salt

1 small head of cauliflower, cut up into small pieces

Half a small red onion and cut it into thin slices

2 cups rice that has been cooked and cooled

1 cup of washed black beans from a can with no added salt

½ cup of chopped queso fresco

1 cup shredded red cabbage

1 medium avocado

1 lime, cut into 4 wedges (Optional)

Directions

Preheat the oven up to 450°F. Put foil around the edges of a big baking sheet with a rim.

In a mixer, blend lime juice, honey, garlic, salt, and chipotles to taste. Process until things are mostly smooth. Put the cauliflower in a big bowl.

Add the sauce and shake it around to coat it. Move to the baking sheet that has been made. Place the onion on top of the cauliflower. It will take 18 to 20 minutes of roasting, turning once, until the cauliflower is soft and browned in spots. Remove from the heat and let it cool.

Put 1/2 cup of quinoa into each of 4 covered dishes that can hold one serving.

On top of each, put a quarter of the cauliflower mix, a quarter cup of black beans, and two tablespoons of cheese. Keep the containers in the fridge for up to 4 days after you seal them.

To warm up one container, open the lid and heat it on high for 2 1/2 to 3 minutes, until it starts to steam.

Add 1/4 cup of cabbage and 1/4 banana (sliced) on top. If you want, you can serve it with a lime wedge.

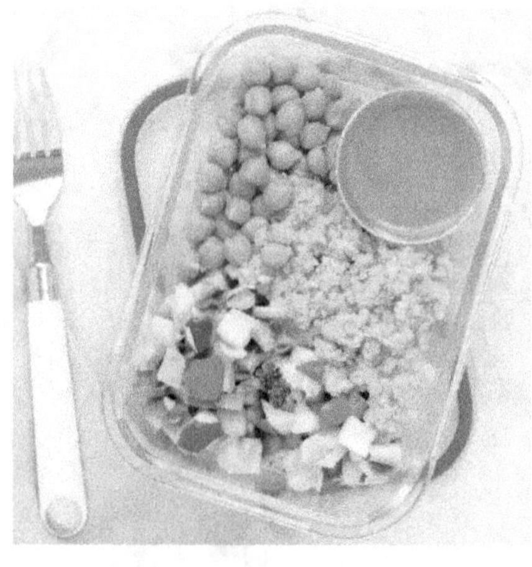

Tip

Look for small cans of smoked chipotle peppers in adobo sauce near other Mexican ingredients in well-stocked supermarkets. Once opened, refrigerate for up to 2 weeks or freeze for up to 6 months.

Nutrition Facts (per serving)

345	Calories
13g	Fat
47g	Carbs
13g	Protein

Chickpea & Potato Curry

Prep Time: 35 mins   **Total Time:** 35 mins

Servings: 4   **Yield:** 5 cups

Ingredients

1 pound Yukon Gold potatoes, peeled and cut into 1-inch pieces

3 tablespoons grapeseed oil or canola oil

1 large onion, diced

3 cloves garlic, minced

2 teaspoons curry powder

¾ teaspoon salt

¼ teaspoon cayenne pepper

1 (14 ounce) can no-salt-added diced tomatoes

¾ cup water, divided

1 (15 ounce) can low-sodium chickpeas, rinsed

1 cup frozen peas

½ teaspoon garam masala (see Tip)

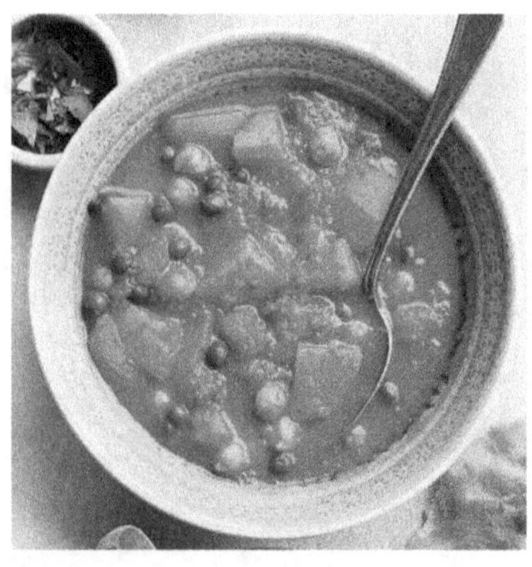

Directions

A large pot with a steamer basket should have an inch of water in it. Bring it to a boil. Cover and steam the potatoes for 6 to 8 minutes, or until they are soft. Leave the potatoes alone. Clean the pot.

Set the pot on medium-high heat and add the oil. For 3 to 5 minutes, turning often, cook the onion until it is soft and clear. Put in the garlic, curry powder, salt, and pepper.

Cook for one minute while stirring all the time. Add the tomato juice and stir. Cook for two minutes. Put the mixture in a food mixer or blender. Blend it with 1/2 cup of water until it is smooth.

Put the mush back in the pot. To get rid of the sauce leftovers, pulse the last 1/4 cup of water in the blender or food processor.

Add the beans, peas, and garam masala to the pot along with the potatoes you saved. For about 5 minutes, stir the food often until it's hot.

Tips

Garam masala, a mix of coriander, black pepper, cumin, cardamom, cinnamon and other spices, adds a warming, complex layer of flavor to this Indian stew.

Nutrition Facts (per serving)

321	Calories
12g	Fat
47g	Carbs
9g	Protein

Falafel Burgers

Prep Time: 30 mins   **Additional Time:** 30 mins   **Total Time:** 1 hr

Servings: 4   **Yield:** 4 servings

Ingredients

½ cup coarsely chopped onion

3 cloves garlic, crushed

1 medium jalapeño pepper, seeded and coarsely chopped

¾ cup fresh cilantro and/or parsley leaves

1 (15 ounce) can no-salt-added chickpeas, rinsed

2 teaspoons ground cumin

1 teaspoon ground coriander

¼ teaspoon baking soda

¼ teaspoon salt

⅓ cup dry whole-wheat breadcrumbs or gluten-free breadcrumbs

1 tablespoon extra-virgin olive oil

4 whole-wheat or gluten-free burger buns, split and toasted

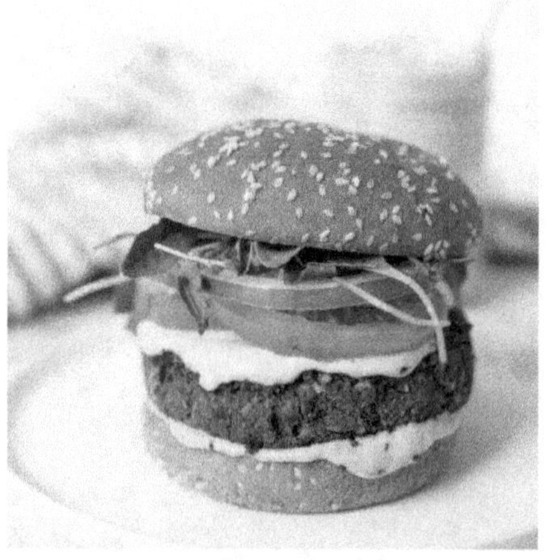

Directions

In a food processor, chop the onion, garlic, jalapeño, and cilantro (or parsley) into small pieces that are all the same size. Spices like cumin, cilantro, baking soda, and salt should be added.

Mix until everything is well mixed. Move to a medium-sized bowl. Put in the breadcrumbs. For 20 minutes, cover and put in the fridge. (This lets the breadcrumbs soak up extra water.)

Warm the oven up to 375 degrees F. using a full 1/3 cup of the chickpea mixture for each patty, make four patties that are 3 inches across.

Put oil in a big pan and set it over medium heat. They should be cooked for about 4 minutes on each side until they are golden and crispy. Carefully move the patties to a baking sheet.

Bake for about 15 minutes, or until warm through and slightly puffed. Put the patties on buns and serve.

Nutrition Facts (per serving)

267	Calories
7g	Fat
43g	Carbs
10g	Protein

Easy Pea & Spinach Carbonara

Prep Time: 20 mins **Total Time:** 20 mins

Servings: 4 **Yield:** 4 cups

Ingredients

1 ½ tablespoons extra-virgin olive oil

½ cup panko breadcrumbs, preferably whole-wheat

1 small clove garlic, minced

8 tablespoons grated Parmesan cheese, divided

3 tablespoons finely chopped fresh parsley

3 large egg yolks

1 large egg

½ teaspoon ground pepper

¼ teaspoon salt

1 (9 ounce) package fresh tagliatelle or linguine

8 cups baby spinach

1 cup peas (fresh or frozen)

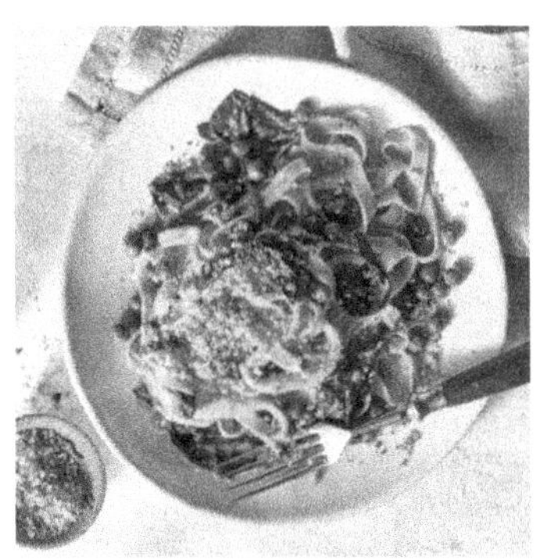

Directions

In a big pot, add 10 cups of water and heat it up until it boils.

At the same time, heat oil in a big pan over medium-high heat. Add the garlic and breadcrumbs.

Cook, turning often, for about two minutes, until the breadcrumbs are golden. Add 2 tablespoons of Parmesan and parsley to a small bowl and mix them in. Put away.

In a medium bowl, mix the egg whites, pepper, salt, and the last 6 tablespoons of Parmesan.

While the water is boiling, cook the pasta for one minute, stirring every now and then.

After you add the spinach and peas, cook for another minute or until the pasta is soft. Keep 1/4 cup of the cooking water aside. Put the rice in a big bowl after draining it.

Slowly whisk the hot water that you saved into the egg mixture. Add the sauce to the pasta slowly, tossing it with tongs to mix. Serve with the breadcrumb mixture that you saved on top.

Nutrition Facts (per serving)

430	Calories
15g	Fat
54g	Carbs

20g   Protein

SOUPS AND STEWS

Hearty Tomato Soup with Beans & Greens

Prep Time: 10 mins   **Total Time:** 10 mins

Servings: 4   **Yield:** 5 cups

Ingredients

2 (14 ounce) cans low-sodium hearty-style tomato soup

1 tablespoon olive oil

3 cups chopped kale

1 teaspoon minced garlic

⅛ teaspoon crushed red pepper (Optional)

1 (14 ounce) can no-salt-added cannellini beans, rinsed

¼ cup grated Parmesan cheese

Directions

Follow the steps on the package to heat the soup in a medium saucepan; simmer over low heat while you prepare the kale.

Put oil in a big pan and set it over medium heat. Stir the kale in and cook for one to two minutes, until it softens. If you want, you can add crushed red pepper and garlic and cook for 30 seconds.

After adding the beans and greens to the soup, let it cook for two to three minutes, or until the beans are warm all the way through.

Put some soup in each of the 4 bowls. Add Parmesan on top and serve.

Nutrition Facts (per serving)

200	Calories
6g	Fat

29g	Carbs	9g	Protein

Stuffed Cabbage Soup

Prep Time: 20 mins   **Additional Time:** 40 mins   **Total Time:** 1 hr

Servings: 8   **Yield:** 8 servings

Ingredients

2 tablespoons of canola oil

1 ½ pounds of lean ground beef

4 cups of chopped green cabbage

2 cups of chopped yellow onion

1 ¼ cups of chopped carrots

1 cup of chopped celery

2 tablespoons of light brown sugar

1 tablespoon of smoked paprika

1 teaspoon of salt

1/8 teaspoon of ground pepper

1/8 teaspoon of cayenne pepper

1 15-ounce can of tomato sauce with no added salt

4 cups of chicken broth without salt

1/2 cup of medium-grain brown rice

2 tablespoons of chopped fresh flat-leaf parsley

Directions

In a big, heavy pot, heat the oil over medium-high heat. Add the ground beef and stir it around a lot. Cook for 6 to 7 minutes, or until the meat is fully cooked and beginning to brown.

Put in the cabbage, onion, carrots, and celery. Cook, turning often, for about 5 minutes, or until the onion is clear.

To the meat mixture, add the brown sugar, paprika, salt, pepper, and cayenne. Stir the spices around constantly over medium-high heat for about one minute, until they smell toasty.

Add the tomato sauce and broth and stir them in. Use a wooden spoon to scrape the bottom of the pot to get rid of any brown bits. Over medium-high heat, bring the soup to a boil. Add the rice and stir.

Turn down the heat, cover, and cook for 30 to 35 minutes, until the rice is soft. If you want, you can add parsley on top before serving.

Nutrition Facts (per serving)

300	Calories

17g	Fat	20g	Protein
18g	Carbs		

Beef & Potato Stew

Active Time: 45 mins   **Total Time:** 3 hrs 45 mins

Servings: 8

Ingredients

3 pounds boneless beef chuck roast, cut into 1 1/2-inch pieces

1 ½ teaspoons salt, divided

1 teaspoon ground pepper

2 tablespoons extra-virgin olive oil

2 medium onions, chopped

8 cloves garlic, peeled and smashed

¼ cup unsalted tomato paste

1 tablespoon chopped fresh rosemary

¼ cup all-purpose flour

2 cups dry red wine, such as cabernet sauvignon

4 cups unsalted beef broth

5 fresh thyme sprigs

1 bay leaf

1 (24 ounce) package baby Yukon Gold potatoes, halved

3 medium carrots, peeled and cut diagonally (1-inch)

2 tablespoons balsamic vinegar

1 tablespoon prepared horseradish

Chopped fresh parsley for garnish

Directions

Put the rack in the bottom third of the oven and heat it up to 325°F. Warm up a big Dutch pot that can go in the oven over medium-high heat.

In a big bowl, mix meat with pepper and 1 teaspoon of salt. Pour oil into the pot and stir it around to cover it.

Pour in the meat in three groups. Cook for two to three minutes on each side, until browned on both sides. Move the food to a plate. Do it again with the rest of the beef.

Lower the heat to medium and add the garlic and onions. Stir often and cook for about 3 minutes, until the onions are soft and beginning to brown a bit.

Add the tomato paste and rosemary. Keep turning the food for about one minute, or until it smells good and the tomato paste turns darker. Add the flour and keep stirring while cooking for about one minute, until the veggies are covered.

Add the wine and bring to a boil. Cook, turning often, for about 5 minutes, or until the sauce is glossy and thick. Add the bay leaf, thyme sprigs, and the last 1/2 teaspoon of salt. Bring to a boil.

Add the beef and any sauces that have built up. Now take it off the heat and put a lid on top of it. Put the dish in the oven and bake for about two hours, or until the sauce has dried out and the beef is mostly soft.

Take the pan out of the oven and add the potatoes and carrots. It will take about an hour of baking with the lid on until the beef, potatoes, and carrots are soft.

Stir in vinegar and horseradish. Decorate with parsley, if desired.

Nutrition Facts (per serving)

435	Calories
11g	Fat
30g	Carbs
42g	Protein

Quick Beef & Barley Soup

Cook Time: 40 mins   **Total Time:** 40 mins

Servings: 4   **Yield:** 4 servings, about 1 1/2 cups each

Ingredients

8 ounces sirloin steak, trimmed and cut into bite-size pieces

½ teaspoon freshly ground pepper, divided

4 teaspoons extra-virgin olive oil, divided

1 medium onion, chopped

1 large stalk celery, sliced

1 large carrot, sliced

2 tablespoons tomato paste

1 tablespoon chopped fresh thyme

¾ cup quick-cooking barley

4 cups reduced-sodium beef broth

1 cup water

¼ teaspoon salt

1-2 teaspoons red-wine vinegar

Directions

Add 1/4 teaspoon of pepper to the steak. Put 2 teaspoons of oil in a Dutch oven and set it over medium heat. Add the steak and stir it around a lot for about two minutes, until it's cooked on all sides. Put it in a bowl.

Adding the last two teaspoons of oil, the onion, and the celery to the pot and moving them around will help them start to soften in about two minutes. Stir the food for two more minutes after adding the carrot. Spread the thyme and tomato paste over the veggies and stir them around. Cook for one to two minutes, until the vegetables are covered in the tomato paste and start to turn brown.

Bring the barley, broth, water, salt, and the last 1/4 teaspoon of pepper to a simmer after adding them. Lower the heat so that it stays at a boil. Cook for about 15 minutes, or until the barley is soft. After a while, add the beef and any extra juices back to the pot. Heat everything through for one to two minutes. Take it off the heat and add vinegar until it tastes right.

Nutrition Facts (per serving)

273	Calories
9g	Fat

| 29g | Carbs | 20g | Protein |

Winter Vegetable Mulligatawny Soup

Active Time: 25 mins   **Total Time:** 50 mins

Servings: 4

Ingredients

1 medium onion, chopped up;

2 medium carrots, chopped up

1 medium parsnip, peeled and chopped up

3 tablespoons extra-virgin olive oil, split

4 cups of diced acorn or butternut squash that has been peeled

1 medium green apple, peeled and finely chopped

1 tablespoon curry powder

3 cloves garlic, minced, divided

1 teaspoon grated fresh ginger

4 cups low-sodium vegetable broth

1 (14 ounce) can no-salt-added diced tomatoes

½ cup red lentils, picked over and rinsed

2 whole-wheat naan flatbreads, halved

¼ cup chopped fresh cilantro, plus more for garnish

Directions

Preheat the oven up to 375°F. Put foil on a baking sheet. In a big saucepan, heat 2 tablespoons of oil over medium-low heat until it swirls. Put in the onion, carrots, and turnip.

Cook for about 6 minutes, or until the onions become clear. Stir in the squash, apple, curry powder, 2 garlic cloves, and ginger. Cook for 1 to 2 minutes, until the food smells good. Mix the beans, tomatoes, and broth together. Bring up the temperature. Turn down the heat to a low level, cover, and cook for about 20 minutes, or until the beans and squash are soft.

In the meantime, use the last tablespoon of oil to brush one side of each bun. Cover with the last garlic clove and place on the baking sheet that has been prepared. Warm it up in the oven for 5 to 6 minutes. Take it out of the oven and sprinkle cilantro on top.

To get the texture you want, mash some of the soup gently with a potato masher. You could also put half of the soup in a blender and mix it until it is smooth. (Be careful when you mix hot liquids.) Add cilantro to the soup and serve it with the bread.

Nutrition Facts (per serving)

487	Calories
15g	Fat
76g	Carbs
14g	Protein

White Bean Soup with Pasta

Active Time: 15 mins   **Total Time:** 25 mins

Servings: 6

How to Make White Bean Soup with Pasta

This hearty soup is the perfect winter meal! Here are tips on how to make it:

Use Frozen Mirepoix

Mirepoix is a combination of diced onion, celery and carrots. It's typically used as a flavor base for stocks, soups and stews. For this recipe, we use frozen mirepoix, which is convenient to have on hand and cuts down on prep time. You can make your own mirepoix by dicing onion, celery and carrots in a 2:1:1 ratio—two parts onion, one part celery and one part carrot. Reserve 1 ½ cups of it for this recipe and freeze the rest.

Choose the White Beans

I use cannellini beans for this recipe, but you can use any type of white bean such as navy beans or Great Northern beans. Just make sure to use low-sodium canned white beans.

Cook the Pasta Separately

Cooking the pasta separately prevents it from overcooking and becoming soggy. If you're making this soup in advance, storing the soup and pasta separately keeps the pasta al dente before reheating. You can refrigerate the soup and pasta in separate airtight containers for up to 3 days.

Ingredients

1 tablespoon extra-virgin olive oil

1 ½ cups frozen mirepoix (diced onion, celery and carrot)

2 cloves garlic, minced

1 teaspoon Italian seasoning

1 teaspoon salt

¼ teaspoon crushed red pepper

¼ teaspoon ground pepper

1 28-ounce can no-salt-added diced tomatoes

2 cups low-sodium no-chicken broth *or* chicken broth

1 15-ounce can low-sodium cannellini beans, rinsed

8 ounces small whole-wheat pasta, such as elbows

1 ½ cups frozen cut-leaf spinach

4 tablespoons grated Parmesan cheese

Directions

Bring a big pot of water to a boil.

In a big pot, heat the oil over medium-high heat. Stir the mirepoix in and cook for about 3 minutes, until it gets soft. Stir in the garlic, Italian seasoning, salt, crushed red pepper, and ground pepper.

Cook for about one minute, until the garlic smells good. Bring the soup, beans, tomatoes and their juices to a boil. Turn down the heat to keep the simmer going strong.

Cover and cook for about 10 minutes, stirring every now and then, until the tomatoes start to break down.

While that is going on, cook the pasta for one minute less than the directions say to do it in the bag. Drain.

Add spinach to the soup and mix it in. Add the pasta right before you serve. Add Parmesan on top and serve.

Nutrition Facts (per serving)

277	Calories
5g	Fat
49g	Carbs
12g	Protein

DESSERTS

Low-Sugar Strawberry Rhubarb Crisp

Active Time: 25 mins   **Total Time:** 1 hr. 10 mins

Servings: 6

teaspoon ground ginger

Ingredients

3 cups chopped fresh *or* frozen, thawed and drained rhubarb (about 12 ounces)

2 cups sliced strawberries (about 12 ounces)

3 tablespoons granulated sugar, divided

2 tablespoons cornstarch

Zest of 1 orange

1 teaspoon vanilla extract

1 teaspoon finely chopped ginger

¼ teaspoon fine salt, divided

1 cup rolled oats

¼ cup white whole-wheat, whole-wheat pastry, all-purpose *or* all-purpose gluten-free flour

4 teaspoons unsalted butter *or* vegan butter, melted

2 tablespoons plus 2 teaspoons canola oil *or* other mild-flavored oil such grapeseed *or* safflower

Directions

Preheat the oven to 350°F. Mix the rhubarb, strawberries, 2 tablespoons of sugar, cornstarch, orange rind, vanilla, ginger, and 1/8 teaspoon of salt in a large bowl.

Pour out into a shallow 2-quart baking dish.

In a medium bowl, add the oats, flour, 1 tablespoon sugar, butter, oil, ground ginger, and the 1/8 teaspoon salt. Spoon the crumb mixture over the fruit.

Cook until the fruit is glazed and syrupy, and the topping golden brown, 30 to 35 minutes. Allow to cool on a wire rack for about 10 minutes before serving.

Nutrition Facts (per serving)

213   Calories

10g	Fat
29g	Carbs
3g	Protein

Strawberry-Chocolate Greek Yogurt Bark

Active Time: 10 mins   **Additional Time:** 3 hrs   **Total Time:** 3 hrs 10 mins

Servings: 32   **Yield:** 32 pieces

Ingredients

3 cups whole-milk plain Greek yogurt

¼ cup pure maple syrup or honey

1 teaspoon vanilla extract

1 ½ cups sliced strawberries

¼ cup mini chocolate chips

Directions

Preheat oven to 375 degrees F. Position the rack in the center of the oven.

In a medium bowl whisk yogurt, maple syrup (or honey) and vanilla. Place on the prepared baking sheet and spread into a 10-by-15-inch rectangle.

Arrange the strawberries on top and then sprinkle chocolate chips all over.

Chill until extremely solid, for at least 3 hours. To serve, cut or break into 32 pieces.

Nutrition Facts (per serving)

34	Calories
1g	Fat
4g	Carbs
2g	Protein

Diabetes-Friendly Carrot Cake

Active Time: 45 mins   **Additional Time:** 25 mins   **Total Time:** 1 hr 10 mins

Servings: 14   **Yield:** 14 servings

Ingredients

Carrot Cake

1 ½ cups all-purpose flour

⅔ cup flax-seed meal

2 teaspoons baking powder

1 teaspoon pumpkin pie spice

½ teaspoon baking soda

¼ teaspoon salt

3 cups finely shredded carrot (about 6 medium carrots) (see Tip)

1 cup refrigerated or frozen egg product, thawed, or 4 eggs, lightly beaten

½ cup granulated sugar (see Tip)

½ cup packed brown sugar (see Tip)

½ cup canola oil

1 Coarsely shredded carrot

Fluffy Cream Cheese Frosting

2 ounces softened reduced-fat cream cheese (Neufchâtel)

½ teaspoon vanilla

¼ cup powdered sugar

1 ½ cups frozen light-whipped dessert topping

Directions

Preheat the oven up to 350°F. To get two 8- or 9-inch round cake pans ready, grease them and dust them with flour.

Put wax paper or parchment paper on the bottom of each pan. Warm the oven up to 350 degrees F. The sides of the pans and waxed or parchment paper should be greased and floured. Put away.

Put the flour, flax seed meal, baking powder, pumpkin pie spice, baking soda, and salt in a big bowl.

Mix them all together, then set them aside. Put the finely chopped carrot, eggs, white sugar, brown sugar, and oil in another big bowl. Mix the ingredients together. Pour the egg mix into the flour mix all at once.

Mix everything together. Spread out an equal amount of batter in each of the pans that have been prepped.

For 8-inch cakes, bake for 25 to 30 minutes. For 9-inch cakes, bake for 20 to 25 minutes, or until a toothpick placed near the middle of the cakes comes out clean.

After the cakes are cool, take them out of the pans and set them on wire racks for 10 minutes. Place the cakes on wire racks while they are upside down. Cool down completely.

Using an electric mixer on medium to high, beat the Neufchâtel and low-fat cream cheese in a medium bowl until the cheese is smooth.

Mix in the vanilla. Sift the powdered sugar in slowly and keep beating the frosting until it is smooth. Let 1.5 cups of frozen light whipped cream topping thaw. About ½ cup of the topping should be mixed into the cream cheese mixture to make it thinner. Next, add the rest of the cream topping and mix it in.

It's time to serve. Put one of the cooled pieces on a plate. On top of the cake, spread half of the Fluffy Cream Cheese Frosting.

Spread the rest of the frosting on top of the second cake layer after putting it on top of the frosting. You could add finely grated carrots if you wanted to.

Tip

When substituting granulated sugar with a sugar substitute, select Splenda Sugar Blend for Baking. In lieu of brown sugar, opt for Splenda Brown Sugar Blend for baking. To utilize the product in a quantity that is equivalent to 1/2 cup of granulated and brown sugars, adhere to the instructions on the package. Nutrition analysis per serving: identical to that provided below, with the exception of 231 calories, 25 grams of carbohydrates, and 186 milligrams of sodium. Calcium constitutes three percent of the recommended daily intake. Exchanges: 1 1/2 other carbohydrates. Carbohydrate alternatives: 1 1/2.

Nutrition Facts (per serving)

254	Calories
12g	Fat
34g	Carbs
5g	Protein

Banana-Bran Muffins

Prep Time: 15 mins   **Active Time:** 15 mins   **Additional Time:** 15 mins

Total Time: 45 mins   **Servings:** 12   **Yield:** 1 dozen muffins

Ingredients

2 large eggs

⅔ cup packed light brown sugar

1 cup mashed ripe bananas, (2 medium)

1 cup buttermilk, (see Ingredient notes)

1 cup unprocessed wheat bran, (see Ingredient notes)

¼ cup canola oil

1 teaspoon vanilla extract

1 cup whole-wheat flour

¾ cup all-purpose flour

1 ½ teaspoons baking powder

½ teaspoon baking soda

½ teaspoon ground cinnamon

¼ teaspoon salt

½ cup chocolate chips (optional)

⅓ cup chopped walnuts (optional)

Directions

Preheat the oven up to 400°F. Spray cooking spray inside 12 muffin tins.

Beat the eggs and brown sugar together in a bowl until the mixture is smooth like paste.

Add the oil, vanilla, buttermilk, and wheat bran, and mix them in. Put all-purpose flour, cinnamon, salt, baking powder, and baking soda in a big bowl.

Mix in the whole-wheat flour. Make a hole in the middle of the dry parts.

Add the wet parts and mix them with the rubber spoon until they are moist. You can add the chocolate chips now if you want to. The muffin cups will be full to the brim when you pour the batter into them. Add walnuts on top if you want to.

Bake the muffins for about 15 to 25 minutes, or until the tops are golden brown and the sides are just a little crispy.

About 5 minutes should pass after baking for the biscuits to cool down in the pan.

Nutrition Facts (per serving)

200	Calories
6g	Fat

| 34g | Carbs |
| 5g | Protein |

Peanut Butter-Oat Energy Balls

Prep Time: 15 mins   **Additional Time:** 15 mins   **Total Time:** 30 mins

Servings: 12   **Yield:** 12 balls

Ingredients

¾ cup chopped Medjool dates

½ cup rolled oats

¼ cup natural peanut butter

Chia seeds for garnish

Directions

Soften dates in warm water for about 5-10 minutes. Drain.

Put the dates, oats and peanut butter into the food processor and blend until the ingredients are very small.

Shape into 12 balls (a scant tablespoon each). Optional, but serve topped with chia seeds. Chill for at least fifteen minutes and up to 1 week.

Nutrition Facts (per serving)

73	Calories
3g	Fat
10g	Carbs
2g	Protein

No-Sugar-Added Vegan Oatmeal Cookies

Prep Time: 25 mins   **Additional Time:** 50 mins   **Total Time:** 1 hr 15 mins

Servings: 12   **Yield:** 2 dozen cookies

Ingredients

1 cup quick-cooking oats (see Tip)

¾ cup almond flour or almond meal

¾ teaspoon ground cinnamon

¼ teaspoon salt

2 medium ripe bananas, mashed

½ cup almond butter or natural peanut butter

1 teaspoon vanilla extract

¾ cup raisins or chopped dates

Directions

Heat the oven to 350 degrees F. Place a large baking sheet ready for use and cover it with parchment paper or a silicone baking mat.

In a large bowl, combine whisked oats, almond flour (or almond meal), cinnamon and salt.

In a large mixing bowl, combine mashed bananas, almond butter (or peanut butter) and vanilla until smooth and thoroughly mixed.

Mix in the dry ingredients and the raisins or dates into the banana mixture using a wooden spoon.

Using tablespoons, scoop or roll the dough into balls and place on the baking sheet lined with parchment paper, to yield 12 cookies per batch. Press gently with a fork to flatten a bit.

Bake until firm to the touch and light brown on the bottom, about 15 minutes.

Remove from the baking sheet and transfer to a wire rack to cool to room temperature completely. Do the same with the rest of the batter.

Tips

Individuals with celiac disease or gluten sensitivity should consume oats that are designated as "gluten-free," as they are frequently cross-contaminated with wheat and barley.

Nutrition Facts (per serving)

177	Calories
10g	Fat
20g	Carbs
5g	Protein

Apple Crumble with Oats

Prep Time: 20 mins   **Additional Time:** 40 mins   **Total Time:** 1 hr

Servings: 6   **Yield:** 6 servings

Ingredients

½ cup regular rolled oats

2 tablespoons whole-wheat pastry flour

2 tablespoons packed brown sugar (see Tips)

½ teaspoon ground cinnamon

1 tablespoon cold butter, cut into small pieces

3 medium Golden Delicious apples, cored and cut into thin wedges

2 tablespoons water

1 tablespoon fresh lemon juice

1 tablespoon packed brown sugar (see Tips)

1 (8 ounce) container Frozen yogurt or low-fat vanilla yogurt

Directions

Preheat the oven up to 350 degrees F. Add the oats, flour, 2 tablespoons of brown sugar, and cinnamon to a medium-sized bowl.

Mix them together. Use a fork to mix it all together. Add the butter and mix it in with your hands, a fork, or a pastry cutter until the dough looks like big crumbs.

Put the apples, water, lemon juice, and the last tablespoon of brown sugar in a big bowl. Put the apple mix into a pie plate that is 9 inches across.

Spread the oat mixture out on top of the apples. At this point, bake for forty to fifty minutes, or until the apple slices are soft and the topping is golden brown. You can warm the mix up and serve it with a yogurt spoon if you want to.

Tips

To make individual servings, prepare as above, except divide the apple mixture among six 6- to 8-ounce custard cups or ramekins. Sprinkle with oat mixture and bake for about 35 minutes or until apples are tender. Serve as above.

If using a sugar substitute, use Splenda(R) Brown Sugar Blend for Baking. Follow package directions to use product amount that's equivalent to 2 and 1 tablespoon brown sugar.

Nutrition Facts (per serving)

148	Calories
3g	Fat
30g	Carbs
3g	Protein

Crispy Peanut Butter Balls

Prep Time: 15 mins   **Additional Time:** 30 mins   **Total Time:** 45 mins

Servings: 12   **Yield:** 12 servings

Ingredients

½ cup natural peanut butter, almond butter or sunflower seed butter

¾ cup crispy rice cereal

1 teaspoon pure maple syrup

½ cup dark chocolate chips, melted (see Tip)

Directions

Place a piece of parchment or wax paper on a baking sheet. Mix together peanut butter, cereal and maple syrup in a bowl.

Divide the mixture into twelve portions, using about 2 teaspoons for each.

Arrange on the prepared baking sheet. Freeze the balls until the balls firm up, approximately 15 minutes.

Coat the balls with the melted chocolate. Return to the freezer until the chocolate is hard, approximately 15 minutes.

Tips

Microwave the chocolate on Medium for one minute to temper it. Stir, and then continue to microwave on Medium, stirring every 20 seconds, until the mixture is melted. Alternatively, position the chocolate in the upper portion of a double boiler that is set over hot water that is not yet boiling. Stir until the substance has completely liquefied.

Nutrition Facts (per serving)

112	Calories
8g	Fat
8g	Carbs
3g	Protein

Peanut Butter Chocolate Chip Cookies

Prep Time: 15 mins   **Additional Time:** 30 mins   **Total Time:** 45 mins

Servings: 15   **Yield:** 30 cookies

Ingredients

1 large egg

¼ teaspoon salt

1 cup smooth natural peanut butter

½ cup light brown sugar

⅓ cup semisweet chocolate chips

Directions

Position rack in middle of oven; preheat to 375 degrees F. Line 2 baking sheets with parchment paper. In a medium bowl, beat the egg with the salt. Mix in peanut butter, brown sugar and chocolate chips into the dough. Using slightly rounded tablespoons, drop the dough about two inches apart on the prepared baking sheets.

Using a fork, flatten each cookie to a 1 3/4-inch diameter by dragging the fork in a crisscross manner. Bake the cookies one sheet at a time until the cookies are just set, 8 to 10 minutes. Allow to set on the pan for 5 minutes before transferring to a wire rack to cool for approximately 20 minutes. Do the same with the rest of cookies.

Nutrition Facts (per serving)

159	Calories
10g	Fat
12g	Carbs
4g	Protein

Crumble Topping

Cook Time: 10 mins   **Total Time:** 10 mins

Servings: 1   **Yield:** 12 individual crumbles or 1 large (9-by-13-inch) crum

Ingredients

1 ½ cups old-fashioned rolled oats

3/4 cup pecans, or almonds, chopped

½ cup brown sugar

1/3 cup whole-wheat flour, or all-purpose flour

¾ teaspoon ground cinnamon

5 tablespoons canola oil

Directions

Mix oats, nuts, brown sugar, flour, and cinnamon in a bowl and blend the mixture until required consistency is attained.

Pour oil on the dry ingredients and mix until all the dry ingredients are wet.

Nutrition Facts (per serving)

159	Calories
10g	Fat
18g	Carbs
2g	Protein

SMOOTHIES

Pineapple Green Smoothie

Active Time: 5 mins   **Total Time:** 5 mins

Servings: 1   **Yield:** 1 serving

Ingredients

½ cup unsweetened almond milk

⅓ cup nonfat plain Greek yogurt

1 cup baby spinach

1 cup frozen banana slices (about 1 medium banana)

½ cup frozen pineapple chunks

1 tablespoon chia seeds

1-2 teaspoons pure maple syrup or honey (optional)

Directions

Add almond milk and yogurt to a blender, then add spinach, banana, pineapple, chia seeds and sweetener (if using); blend until smooth.

Tips

You may (or may not) want your smoothie a little sweeter. Since both bananas and pineapple can vary in sweetness, I recommend keeping the added sugar optional and adding it only after you're sure your smoothie needs it.

After all, it's easier to add sugar than it is to take it away! Start with a teaspoon, and add more to taste. I recommend adding liquid sweeteners like pure maple syrup or honey.

Nutrition Facts (per serving)

297	Calories
6g	Fat
54g	Carbs
13g	Protein

Strawberry-Blueberry-Banana Smoothie

Prep Time: 5 mins   **Total Time:** 5 mins

Servings: 1   **Yield:** 2 cups

Ingredients

½ cup frozen strawberries

½ cup frozen blueberries

1 small ripe banana (frozen, if desired)

¾ cup chilled unsweetened cashew milk, plus more if needed

1 tablespoon cashew butter

1 tablespoon hulled hemp seeds

Directions

Combine strawberries, blueberries, banana, cashew milk, cashew butter and hemp seeds in a blender.

Process until smooth, adding more cashew milk, if needed, for desired consistency. Serve immediately.

Nutrition Facts (per serving)

335	Calories
17g	Fat
46g	Carbs
7g	Protein

Really Green Smoothie

Prep Time: 5 mins   **Total Time:** 5 mins

Servings: 1   **Yield:** 1 serving

Ingredients

1 large ripe banana

1 cup packed baby kale or coarsely chopped mature kale

1 cup unsweetened vanilla almond milk

¼ ripe avocado

1 tablespoon chia seeds

2 teaspoons honey

1 cup ice cubes

Directions

Combine banana, kale, almond milk, avocado, chia seeds and honey in a blender. Blend on high until creamy and smooth. Add ice and blend until smooth.

Nutrition Facts (per serving)

343	Calories
14g	Fat
55g	Carbs
6g	Protein

Anti-Inflammatory Lemon-Blueberry Smoothie

Active Time: 5 mins   **Total Time:** 5 mins

Servings: 1 serving

Ingredients

1 cup frozen blueberries, plus more for garnish

1 medium ripe banana, peeled and frozen

1 cup packed baby kale

1/2 cup unsweetened plain almond milk

1/2 cup chilled unsweetened brewed green tea

2 tablespoons hulled hemp seeds

3/4 teaspoon lemon zest, plus more for garnish

1 1/2 tablespoons lemon juice

1/2 teaspoon honey (optional)

1/4 teaspoon ground ginger

Directions

Place blueberries, banana, kale, almond milk, tea, hemp seeds, lemon zest, lemon juice, honey (if using) and ginger in a blender; process until smooth, about 25 seconds.

Pour into a glass. Garnish with additional blueberries and/or lemon zest, if desired.

Nutrition Facts (per serving)

330	Calories
13g	Fat
52g	Carbs
10g	Protein

Strawberry-Chocolate Smoothie

Prep Time: 5 mins   **Total Time:** 5 mins

Servings: 1   **Yield:** 2 cups

Ingredients

1 ½ cups frozen strawberries

1 cup chilled unsweetened chocolate almond milk, plus more if needed

1 tablespoon almond butter

1 tablespoon unsweetened cocoa powder

1 tablespoon honey

Directions

Combine strawberries, almond milk, almond butter, cocoa and honey in a blender.

Process until smooth, adding more almond milk, if needed, for desired consistency. Serve immediately.

Nutrition Facts (per serving)

303	Calories
13g	Fat
47g	Carbs
7g	Protein

SIDES

This Roasted Cabbage Salad with Lemon-Garlic Vinaigrette Is "Super Tasty"

Active Time: 10 mins   **Total Time:** 50 mins

Servings: 6

Ingredients

Olive oil cooking spray

1 medium head cabbage

1/2 teaspoon salt, divided

Ground pepper to taste

1/4 cup extra-virgin olive oil

1 1/2 tablespoons red-wine vinegar

1 tablespoon lemon juice

1 1/2 teaspoons Dijon mustard

1 small clove garlic, grated

2 tablespoons sliced almonds, toasted (see Tip)

2 tablespoons minced fresh chives *or* parsley

Directions

Preheat oven to 400°F. Prepare a large baking sheet with aluminum foil, parchment paper or a silicone baking sheet; lightly spray with olive oil cooking spray.

Discard outer leaves of cabbage and cut into 8 sections while keeping root end intact. Place the wedges in the prepared pan. Lightly grease the tops of the wedges with cooking spray and sprinkle with ¼ teaspoon salt and pepper.

Cook the cabbage on the back side of the pan, and turn the wedges over halfway through, until caramelized and tender, for about 30 to 40 minutes.

At the same time, in a sealable jar, whisk together the oil, vinegar, lemon juice, mustard, garlic, ¼ teaspoon salt and black pepper. Mix well and then cover before shaking.

Allow the cabbage to stand for 5 minutes then chop it roughly. Transfer to a shallow serving dish and pour the dressing over the rice. Top with almonds and chives (or parsley) before serving.

Tip

For the best flavor, toast nuts before using in a recipe. To toast sliced nuts, place in a small dry skillet and cook over medium-low heat, stirring constantly, until fragrant, 2 to 4 minutes.

Nutrition Facts (per serving)

132	Calories
13g	Fat
5g	Carbs
1g	Protein

Crispy Smashed Beets with Goat Cheese

Prep Time: 30 mins   **Additional Time:** 1 hr 30 mins   **Total Time:** 2 hrs

Servings: 4   **Yield:** 4 servings

Ingredients

6 small or 4 medium beets (about 1 pound), trimmed and either scrubbed or peeled

¼ cup balsamic vinegar

2 sprigs fresh rosemary

¼ cup goat cheese (2 ounces), at room temperature

2 tablespoons milk

2 tablespoons snipped fresh chives

Pinch plus 1/4 teaspoon salt, divided

Pinch plus 1/4 teaspoon ground pepper, divided

2 tablespoons extra-virgin olive oil, divided

Directions

Put beets, vinegar and rosemary together in one layer in a large saucepan. Pour water on the mixture such that it covers it by about two inches.

Boil, then lower the heat and let the mixture simmer. Place the lid on and cook until the beets are soft, about 1 to 1 1/2 hours.

At the same time, in a separate bowl, combine goat cheese and milk until you get a smooth mixture. Add chives and sprinkle with salt and pepper to taste. Allow to stand at ambient temperature.

Once the beets are tender, turn off the heat and, using a slotted spoon, transfer the beets to a cutting board. To prepare beets cut each beet in half vertically.

Gently tamp each beet with a large dinner plate or a mason jar so that it barely holds together. Season both sides of the beets with the remaining 1/4 teaspoon salt and pepper. Heat 1 tablespoon oil in a large skillet over medium-high heat.

Mix half of the beets and fry, flipping once, until golden on the outside and crunchy throughout, 3 to 6 minutes in total. Transfer to a plate.

Pour the remaining 1 tablespoon oil into the pan and sauté the other beets in the same manner.

Accompany with a spoonful of the goat cheese mixture.

Nutrition Facts (per serving)

170   Calories

11g   Fat

14g   Carbs

5g   Protein

Brussels sprouts Caesar Salad

Active Time: 25 mins   **Total Time:** 25 mins

Servings: 4

Ingredients

2 tablespoons canola oil

1 pound medium Brussels sprouts, trimmed and halved lengthwise

2 teaspoons grated lemon zest

2 tablespoons lemon juice

1 tablespoon mayonnaise

1 small clove garlic, finely chopped

1 teaspoon white-wine vinegar

1 teaspoon Worcestershire sauce

1/2 teaspoon ground pepper

4 tablespoons grated Parmesan cheese, divided

2 cups chopped romaine lettuce hearts

1/2 cup Caesar-seasoned croutons, coarsely chopped

Directions

Heat the oven to 425 degrees Fahrenheit. Heat oil in a large cast-iron skillet over medium-high heat until it begins the process of smoking.

Place Brussels sprouts with the cut side on the bottom; cook without turning, until the bottoms are well-browned, 4 to 5 minutes.

Flip Brussels sprouts. Transfer to the oven; roast until browned on edges and tender-crisp, 6 to 8 minutes. Let cool slightly, about 5 minutes.

Meanwhile, whisk lemon zest, lemon juice, mayonnaise, garlic, vinegar, Worcestershire, pepper and 3 tablespoons Parmesan together in a large bowl until smooth.

Add the Brussels sprouts, romaine and croutons; toss until evenly coated.

Divide among 4 plates; sprinkle evenly with the remaining 1 tablespoon Parmesan.

Nutrition Facts (per serving)

204	Calories
13g	Fat
19g	Carbs
8g	Protein

Hot Honey Parmesan Carrots

Active Time: 10 mins   **Total Time:** 35 mins

Servings: 4

Ingredients

1 1/2 pounds carrots, peeled

1/3 cup finely grated Parmesan cheese

1 tablespoon extra-virgin olive oil

1/2 teaspoon granulated garlic

1/2 teaspoon onion powder

1/8 teaspoon salt

1 tablespoon hot honey

Directions

Preheat oven to 400°F. Prepare carrots to measure 1 1/2 inches on the cross-section. Slice each piece in half lengthwise; arrange in a medium bowl.

Toss well the carrots with Parmesan, oil, garlic, onion powder and salt. Spread out the carrots, with the cut sides down, in a single layer on a large baking sheet with a rim.

Roast in the oven until the carrots are soft and cheese is brown and crunchy, approximately 25-30min.

Put the carrots into a serving dish. Pour hot honey over it in an even manner.

Nutrition Facts (per serving)

153	Calories
6g	Fat
22g	Carbs
4g	Protein

Fennel & Grapefruit Salad

Prep Time: 15 mins   **Total Time:** 15 mins

Servings: 4   **Yield:** 4 cups

Ingredients

1 large grapefruit

1 teaspoon honey

1 teaspoon Dijon mustard

¼ teaspoon salt

⅛ teaspoon ground pepper

1 tablespoon plus 1 teaspoon canola oil

1 small fennel bulb, cored and thinly sliced, plus fennel fronds for garnish

1 medium Granny Smith apple, cored and thinly sliced

1 tablespoon toasted sunflower seeds

Directions

Zest grapefruit into a large bowl until you have 1 tablespoon zest.

Working over a small bowl, cut the grapefruit into segments (see Tip). Cut the segments into thirds; set aside.

Squeeze 2 tablespoons juice from the leftover membranes into the large bowl with the zest.

Add honey, mustard, salt, and pepper to the large bowl; whisk to combine. Whisk in the oil, stirring until fully combined.

Add fennel, apple, and the reserved grapefruit to the bowl and toss until combined. Sprinkle with sunflower seeds. Garnish with fennel fronds, if desired.

Tips

To segment a grapefruit (or orange), slice a small piece off the top and bottom. Slice along the curve of the fruit from top to bottom to remove the peel. Cut each segment from the surrounding membranes.

Nutrition Facts (per serving)

130	Calories
6g	Fat
19g	Carbs
2g	Protein

SNACKS

Roasted Honeynut Squash

Prep Time: 10 mins   **Additional Time:** 30 mins   **Total Time:** 40 mins

Servings: 4   **Yield:** 4 serving

Prepping Honeynut Squash

The squashes are incredibly simple to prepare, and they serve only one to two people each (finally, a squash that we won't be consuming for days!). The process is as follows:

Keep the squash as steady as possible on a chopping board. In a lengthwise trajectory, insert the tip of a large, heavy chef's knife into the center of the squash.

Position a folded kitchen towel between your hand and the knife's spine and apply pressure to guide the knife through one half of the squash. Rotate the squash 180 degrees and repeat the procedure on the opposite side.

Scoop out the seeds and the initial shallow layer of flesh with a utensil to achieve a smoother surface. The seeds may be cleaned and roasted in the same manner as pumpkin seeds, or they may be discarded.

Ingredients

2 medium honeynut squash, halved lengthwise and seeded

4 teaspoons butter

¼ teaspoon salt

¼ teaspoon ground pepper

¼ teaspoon ground cinnamon

4 teaspoons pure maple syrup (optional)

Directions

Preheat the oven to 425°F.

Place the squash halves, cut-side up, on a large, rimmed baking sheet. Place one teaspoon of butter in each cavity.

Sprinkle with cinnamon, salt, and pepper. Roast for 25 to 30 minutes until the meat is tender. Drizzle maple syrup if desired

Nutrition Facts (per serving)

114	Calories
4g	Fat
21g	Carbs
2g	Protein

Roasted Sweet Potatoes

Active Time: 10 mins   **Additional Time:** 20 mins   **Total Time:** 30 mins

Servings: 4   **Yield:** 4 servings

Ingredients

1 pound sweet potatoes (about 2 medium), scrubbed

1 ½ teaspoons olive oil

¼ teaspoon kosher salt

⅛ teaspoon ground pepper

Directions

Preheat oven to 425°F. Place a baking sheet that has edges on a foil; grease it with a cooking spray lightly. Set aside. For the unpeeled sweet potatoes, cut them into one-inch cubes.

Coat sweet potatoes with oil, kosher salt and pepper in a large mixing bowl. Place sweet potatoes on a baking sheet in a single layer. Bake for 20 minutes or until golden brown and crunchy on the scored parts and soft within, flipping once.

Nutrition Facts (per serving)

85	Calories
2g	Fat
17g	Carbs
1g	Protein

Sautéed Butternut Squash

Prep Time: 15 mins   **Additional Time:** 15 mins   **Total Time:** 30 mins

Servings: 7   **Yield:** 7 servings

Ingredients

1 large butternut squash (2-3 pounds), peeled, seeded and cubed

1 tablespoon of extra-virgin olive oil

Directions

In a large saucepan set the heat to medium and add oil.

Stir in squash; cook, stirring occasionally, until the veggies are softened and lightly caramelized, 15–20 minutes.

Tips

To make ahead: Peel and cube squash; refrigerate, covered, for up to 3 days before cooking.

Nutrition Facts (per serving)

75	Calories
2g	Fat
15g	Carbs
1g	Protein

Air-Fryer Sweet Potato Fries

Prep Time: 10 mins   **Additional Time:** 10 mins   **Total Time:** 20 mins

Servings: 4   **Yield:** 4 servings

Ingredients

1 tablespoon olive oil

¼ teaspoon sea salt

¼ teaspoon ground pepper

¼ teaspoon cayenne pepper

¼ teaspoon ground cinnamon

2 medium sweet potatoes, peeled and sliced into 1/4-inch sticks

Directions

Spray an air-fryer basket lightly with cooking spray.

Mix oil, salt, pepper, cayenne and cinnamon in a large bowl. Stir in sweet potatoes; turn to coat well.

Arrange the sweet potatoes in a single layer on the prepared basket. Bake at 400 degrees F until crispy, 14 minutes, turning over halfway through.

Drain the fries on a paper towel to get rid of excess oil. Serve immediately.

Nutrition Facts (per serving)

84	Calories
4g	Fat
12g	Carbs
1g	Protein

Baked Banana-Nut Oatmeal Cups

Prep Time: 15 mins   **Additional Time:** 35 mins   **Total Time:** 50 mins

Servings: 12   **Yield:** 12 muffins

Ingredients

3 cups rolled oats (see Tip)

1 ½ cups low fat milk

2 large ripe bananas, mashed for about three fourth cup.

⅓ cup packed brown sugar

2 large eggs which should be lightly beaten

1 teaspoon baking powder

1 teaspoon ground cinnamon

It is suggested to add 1 teaspoon vanilla extract.

½ teaspoon salt

½ cup chopped toasted pecan nuts

Directions

Preheat oven to 375°F. The next step is to grease a muffin tin with cooking spray.

In a large bowl mix oats, the milk, bananas, brown sugar, eggs, baking powder, cinnamon, vanilla, and salt. Fold in pecans. Spoon the mixture into the muffin cups, filling approximately one-third full. Place the pan in the pre-heated oven and bake for 25 minutes or until a tooth pick inserted in the center of the cake will come out clean. Leave in the pan for 10 minutes before turning the puddings out onto a wire rack to cool. It is best served warm, but it is just as perfect at room temperature.

Tip

It is recommended that individuals with celiac disease or gluten intolerance use oats that are specifically labelled "gluten-free" since oats are usually contaminated with wheat or barley.

Nutrition Facts (per serving)

176	Calories
6g	Fat
26g	Carbs
5g	Protein

CONCLUSION

Thank you for embarking on this culinary journey with **"LOW CHOLESTEROL COOKBOOK FOR BEGINNERS 2024**." As stated above, it is my desire that this book has given you the ability to better manage your heart's health through the foods you cook and eat.

Lowering cholesterol levels is one of the ways towards improving your health and it is encouraging that you are ready to make the necessary changes. The recipes and tips in these pages are aimed at helping you reduce your cholesterol levels and, at the same time, help you live a happier and healthier life through great-tasting, wholesome meals that can be enjoyed with family and friends.

Key Takeaways

- *Understand Cholesterol:* Knowledge is power. To effectively manage your cholesterol levels it is important to comprehend the differences between HDL and LDL cholesterol and their effects on the body.
- *Eat Heart-Healthy Foods:* Increase your consumption of fruits, vegetables, whole grains, lean proteins, and healthy fats in your diet. Reduce intake of foods which are rich in fat especially saturated fats, trans fat and cholesterol.
- *Follow Practical Tips:* Instead, use the following tips to manage cholesterol through diet: Some of them are selecting fiber rich foods, healthy fats, and omega-3 fatty acids.
- *Plan Your Meals:* By following the meal planning guides and recipes here, you can prepare healthy and nutritious meals that are good for your heart. This way, you remain focused and minimize the chances of giving in to foods that you know are not good for you.
- *Monitor Your Progress:* Monitor your cholesterol levels from time to time and visit your doctor or nutritionist for help on the right measures to take regarding diet.

Embrace a Healthier Lifestyle

Eating low cholesterol foods is not a one-time endeavor; it is a lifestyle change. Be proud of your accomplishments, accept failures as lessons, and keep on discovering more recipes and ways towards better diet. Cooking food at home means you can choose what goes into your food and how the food is prepared, and cooking is a step toward a healthy life.

Stay Connected

Bear in mind that you are not on this journey alone. Feel free to describe your experiences, achievements, or even failures to the community of like-minded people. Whether it is in the social networks, in the cooking courses or in the support groups, interaction helps motivate and share new inspirations to make the diet not only interesting, but efficient as well.

Final Thoughts

Healthy eating is not solely about cutting down on certain figures on a chart; it's about improving the quality of life. You are making a wise choice when you decide to take control of your future and your health by eating right. Savor the moments of browsing through cookbooks, taste the new dishes, and feel the benefits of proper nutrition for the body and soul.

Thank you for choosing "LOW CHOLESTEROL COOKBOOK FOR BEGINNERS

2024."

Wishing you good health, joy, and a tasty low cholesterol life!

Wishing you the very best in your journey,

 Verna R. Chapman

I HAVE A REQUEST

Dear Reader,

It's my pleasure to have you onboard. I appreciate your interest and the efforts you've made to change your nutritional habits for the sake of your heart health.

I really appreciate your comments and feedback, as well as your understanding of how this cookbook can be useful to others. If the recipes and information in this book were helpful to you, I would kindly appreciate it if you could leave a comment on the Amazon listing. Just your unadulterated opinion output can go a long way toward helping others stumble on this useful tool.

To leave a review for the book, please go to the Amazon page where you purchased the book and scroll down to the reviews section. Share your experience with the book-What did you like about the book? Which recipes were your favorites? How has the book helped you manage your cholesterol? Do you have any favorite tips or sections? Your detailed feedback not only inspires me but may also help others who are on the same quest to improve their heart health. Writing this cookbook has been a joy, and understanding how it helps improve your health benefits me beyond words.

Thank you for your support, and your feedback fuels me to keep providing information that will help others.

Warm regards,

Verna R. Chapman